Global Patterns of **HIV/AIDS Transmission**

Global Patterns of HIV/AIDS Transmission

Dr. V. Ramamurthy

AUTHORSPRESS

First Published 2000
by Authorspress

E-35/103, Jawahar Park (Shree Ganesh Complex),
Laxmi Nagar, Delhi-110 092
e-mail: authorspress@yahoo.com

Typeset in NewCenturySchlbk by Chitra Computers

Global Patterns of HIV/AIDS Transmission
ISBN 81-7273-018-7

Printed in India at Tarun Offset, Delhi.

Preface

The exact origin of HIV and its introduction to humans is unknown, but there is much speculation and theorising about where and how HIV infection first developed. One proposed explanation for HIV is that it was well established in all areas of the world but has only recently been recognised. However, this theory has not been well substantiated. A second proposition holds that HIV evolved through the mutation of an older and nonpathogenic virus. Virologists, however, have dismissed this as a plausible explanation for HIV on the basis of specific characteristics of the virus and its relationship to other viruses. A third and widely discussed possible origin of HIV is zoonosis, the recent entry of a non-human virus into human populations. This is a plausible explanation for the emergence of HIV because similar viruses exist in old-world apes that live in areas that surround African regions where HIV is endemic. Still, zoonosis has not been universally accepted as the source of HIV. The most widely held view of HIV is that it represents a virus that developed in humans in Central Africa and only recently spread because of social changes, most importantly global travel and transcontinental commerce.

The spread of HIV varies greatly by geographic regions of the world. The World Health Organisation has estimated that over seven million Africans, one million North Americans, one million South Americans, and one million Asians are HIV infected. Differences in epidemiological patterns among continents are striking and lead to disparate rates of disease among men and women, heterosexuals and homosexuals, and infected children. HIV has been primarily spread through male homosexual and bisexual contact and through contaminated injection equipment.

An overwhelming amount of evidence shows that AIDS is the direct result of HIV infection. Although there are several cases of HIV infection and AIDS that remain unclassified with respect to mode of viral transmission, virtually all cases of AIDS are eventually linked to sexual behaviour, injection drug use, or receiving blood or blood products. Despite the fact that HIV is controllable through behaviour changes and that the vast majority of people at risk are aware of how HIV is contracted, the epidemic is expanding at dramatic rates. Worldwide, the HIV epidemic doubles every 1 to 3 years among heterosexually active adults.

Networks of concerned people and organisations that are either international or transnational create a growing capacity for sharing, communication, and solidarity that crosses national boundaries. Global interdependence is a reality that we in health have been rather slow to recognise, and it is bringing about a growing capacity to transcend national borders, to join community activism with a global consciousness and conscience.

Yet there is a tension between the continued relevance of community and national specificity and global thinking. We need not choose among the extremes of tribalism, nationalism, or globalism—yet the future of more than AIDS may depend upon how these tendencies are negotiated. Thus a global epidemic of infectious disease helps us not only to explore health and science, but also to appreciate further forces that are shaping the modern world. The community, national, and international response to the AIDS pandemic mirrors and helps to shape the global future.

Author

Contents

	Preface	v
1.	Impact of AIDS in Society	1
2.	HIV Baby Booms	73
3.	Epidemiology of HIV	93
4.	AIDS and Social Adjustments	118
5.	AIDS and Environmental Stressors	167
6.	Rise of Western AIDS Epidemic	191
7.	AIDS Counselling	207
8.	HIV Transmission through Breast-feeding	267
9.	AIDS: A Challenge for Human Race	283
	Bibliography	301
	Index	308

1

Impact of AIDS in Society

There are many impacts of the AIDS epidemic that cannot be quantified, for example, the emotional pain experienced by infected individuals and their families and the psychological damage wrought on surviving family members. These impacts are very important but how to respond to them is beyond our expertise and best left to others. This chapter considers the economic aspects of three types of impacts—on infected individuals, on the health sector generally and on surviving household members—the ways in which government policies can help people to cope, given the many other pressing demands for scarce public resources.

There are affordable, effective and humane ways for governments in low-income countries to help and ease the suffering of individuals infected with HIV. However, both governments and individuals in the poorest countries should be wary of funding expensive treatments with uncertain benefits.

Health Care for the Person with AIDS

What is the health impact of HIV/AIDS on an infected individual over the course of the disease? Are there effective, affordable treatments for people with AIDS in low-income countries? To answer these questions, this part of the chapter reviews the many illnesses that often afflict people with HIV/AIDS, the available treatments and their cost. It distinguishes between three types of care: relief of symptoms, such as headache, pain, diarrhoea and shortness of breath, which is sometimes called palliative care;

prevention and treatment of opportunistic illnesses (OIs); and antiretroviral (ARV) treatments, which attempt to combat HIV itself. Next it presents the amounts that developing countries are actually spending to care for people with HIV/AIDS. While this amount is often large relative to a country's GNP per capita, it is usually too little to buy all the drugs needed to treat opportunistic illnesses, much less to pay for antiretroviral therapy.

Palliative care

Pattern of opportunistic illnesses differs from country to country, depending on which diseases are prevalent and the quality and amount of treatment available.

In the early stages of HIV illness, palliative treatment can inexpensively relieve some of the pain, discomfort and incontinence that otherwise rob people of the ability to enjoy life and contribute to their family and their community. The opportunistic illnesses that commonly arise early in the course of AIDS can also be treated quite inexpensively. Treatment for thrush, toxoplasmosis and pneumonia/ septicemia can buy one to four years of life at an additional drug cost of $30 to $150—all but the very poor would probably be willing and able to pay for these treatments. Rarer opportunistic illnesses like the fungal diseases tend to occur later in the course of the HIV infection and are more difficult and expensive to treat.

Many of the symptoms and opportunistic illnesses that occur in the early stages of AIDS can be effectively treated at low cost. Unfortunately, the low-cost generic forms of the needed drugs are often unavailable; even when they are available, people often lack information about their efficacy. Governments can address these problems by facilitating the availability of generic drugs needed for palliative care and common opportunistic illnesses.

For example, countries with a concentrated or generalised epidemic could add these medications to their list of "essential drugs," which are widely distributed. Governments can also help patients to make informed decisions by ensuring access to reliable information about the efficacy of various treatment options, both pharmaceuticals and traditional remedies. The degree of government subsidy for treatment will depend on the country's overall health financing policy.

The treatments discussed above ease suffering and prolong life but ultimately fail to save the patient's life because none attacks the underlying cause of illness—the continued spread of HIV within the body and the consequent decline of the immune system's ability to recognise and repel biological threats. A few drugs have reduced the levels of HIV in the patient's blood below the ability of laboratory tests to detect it.

Unfortunately, these drugs are expensive and complex to administer, their long-term benefits are uncertain and their efficacy varies greatly from one individual to another. The first drug that showed evidence of inhibiting the spread of the virus in an infected patient was zidovidine (AZT, or ZDV). When AZT was introduced in the late 1980s, the cost of a year's dosage was about $10,000 in industrial countries. By 1997 the cost of a year's dose had fallen to about $2,738 in industrial countries, while Thailand and a few other developing countries had negotiated bulk purchases for as little as $657 per patient per year. However, except for prevention of mother-to-child transmission, AZT rarely provided dramatic benefits, adding perhaps six months of healthy life for the average patient.

A more effective therapy involving the use of three antiretrovirals was announced in June 1996. A year later, the U.S. government issued draft guidelines recommending early, aggressive treatment of HIV-infected individuals with triple-drug therapy. However, it was clear that more time would be needed before the new therapies could be fully assessed. Some individuals taking the medicines in clinical trials have dramatically improved their health and no longer have detectable levels of viral RNA activity.

Yet even among these patients, the virus may only be hiding and could re-emerge. And other patients show little or no reduction in viral levels, while still others cannot tolerate the drugs. As of mid-1997 no studies had yet been completed estimating the average percentage of patients who could benefit from triple-drug therapy or the characteristics of patients most likely to respond favourably—or to relapse.

Even if the therapy is shown to be generally effective, three substantial problems will remain: the cost of the drugs themselves, the costs and difficulty of the monitoring needed for the therapy to be effective and problems with patient compliance. Although all of these problems also exist in industrial countries, they are likely to be especially severe in developing country medical settings.

Effective antiretroviral therapy requires a highly trained, specialised physician working in a well-equipped clinic with experience performing a wide range of sophisticated tests and procedures, all of which are in critically short supply in most developing countries.

In the event that cost and infrastructure problems could somehow be overcome, patient compliance would continue to pose serious difficulties. Patients undertaking triple-drug therapy must swallow up to 20 pills a day according to a complex schedule related to sleep and meal times. Failure to follow the schedule increases the chance that the virus will become resistant or that the patient will be too sickened by the drugs to continue treatment. Even well-educated patients with good clinical support have difficulty adhering to this demanding regimen; moreover, patients in the early stages of HIV infection are sometimes not willing to take drugs that make them nauseous when they otherwise feel healthy.

In clinical trials in industrial countries, for example, as few as 26 per cent of patients complied with the instructions. Problems with patient compliance are likely to be worse in low-income countries due to lower education levels and the many other problems that poor people in developing countries face. Even with all these difficulties and uncertainties, many patients in developing countries will ask their physicians for triple-drug therapy, just as patients have attempted to obtain AZT. Governments will in turn face pressure to buy these drugs and to subsidize the necessary clinical services. When very few people have

AIDS, total costs will also be small relative to other government expenditures. But as the epidemic progresses, the number of AIDS cases and the cost of the subsidy will escalate rapidly, drawing resources from other pressing social needs.

Alternatives to expensive inpatient care

Where the AIDS epidemic is severe, health policymakers inside and outside government have sought ways to provide compassionate care at low cost. Three alternatives to expensive inpatient care are outpatient AIDS clinics, hospice care (residential low-technology care for the terminally ill) and home-based care. One innovative program to deliver high-quality treatment of symptoms and opportunistic illnesses without the expense of hospitalisation was an outpatient clinic started in 1989 in Sao Paulo, Brazil. Such clinics are especially well suited to serve urban HIV-positive and AIDS patients who are able to leave their homes.

Later in the course of the disease, when the patient is less mobile, the hospice or nursing home provides a lower-cost substitute for inpatient care in a sophisticated referral hospital. However, since such facilities are rarely available in developing countries, the main alternative to the hospital is care at home.

Assuming that the average patient with AIDS would survive six months with either type of care, the benefits of home-based care must be measured in reductions of hospitalisation cost: reduced travel time to the hospital for the patient and the patient's caretakers; increased patient satisfaction and comfort; and ancillary benefits to the community, such as improved understanding of the ways to prevent AIDS and decreased stigma toward HIV-positive people.

A study in Zambia found that patients who received home-based care reduced their hospitalisation before death by only two days, the expenditure on the hospital-initiated home-based care programs of about \$312 (6 months × 2 visits per month × \$26 per visit) was much more than the \$14.50 saving in hospital charges (2 days × \$7.25 per day). On the other hand, the costs for six months of community-initiated home-based care averaged just $26, less than one-tenth the cost of the hospital-initiated program and could almost be justified on the basis of reduced hospital use alone.

The tenfold cost difference between hospital and community initiated home care programs was due to the much larger expenditure on transport and staff time for the hospital-based programs. For example, on a typical day a team of trained hospital-based nurses could visit only four to eight patients, about a quarter of whom were away from home when the team arrived.

If the low cost of the community-initiated home-based care program in Zambia can be generalised to other settings, it is possible that such care would be financed by the patients, their families and their communities. Indeed, the community-initiated Zambian programs function well because of strong volunteer support from the local communities. Since the benefits of the program include the public ones of improved knowledge about HIV prevention and reduced stigma, there may be a government role in financing such programs, at least until their private benefits to patients' families are sufficiently well understood for these families and communities to support such programs on their own.

HEALTH POLICY CHOICES IN A SEVERE 'AIDS EPIDEMIC

Here we discuss the need to keep costs low becomes more apparent as we widen the focus from the individual HIV-infected person to the health care needs of all people in a country. To better understand the difficult tradeoffs involved, we first estimate the magnitude of the impact of AIDS on the health sector and then discuss how government policies can mitigate this impact.

AIDS will affect the health sector in two ways: by increasing demand and by reducing the supply of a given quality of care at a given price. As a result, some HIV-negative people who would have obtained treatment had there been no epidemic will be unable to do so and total national expenditure on health care will rise, both in absolute terms and as a proportion of national product.

Increased demand for care: Most people who develop AIDS are prime-age adults. Without AIDS, this 15-to-50 age group accounts for only 10 to 20 per cent of all deaths in a developing country, but these deaths typically generate a disproportionate share of total health care demand. Moreover, since several studies suggest that adults with AIDS use more health care prior to death than those who die of other causes, or even of other prolonged illnesses, the percentage increase in the demand for care by adults is likely to exceed the percentage increase in their mortality due to AIDS.

As a result of these two factors, in a country where prime-age adults utilised one-quarter of all health care before AIDS, a given percentage increase in their demand for health care will increase total demand by at least one-quarter of that percentage. For example, a 40 per cent increase in the mortality rate of prime-age adults will increase total demand by at least 10 per cent, even though total mortality has increased by only 4 per cent to 8 percent. If AIDS patients use expensive antiretroviral therapies, the increase in demand will be much greater. How much the demand for care increases in the aggregate depends on the increase in the prime-age adult death rate, which in turn depends on the level of HIV prevalence and the median time from infection to death.

A stable prevalence rate of 5 per cent among prime-age adults eventually increases their annual mortality by about five deaths per 1,000 adults if the median time from infection to death is ten years, or by about ten deaths if the median time is only five years.

A prevalence rate of 30 per cent, such as is observed in Lusaka, Zambia, will increase the number of deaths per 1,000 adults by 30 to 60, depending on the median time to death. In Sub-Saharan Africa, where mortality rates in this age group were as high as five per 1,000 before the epidemic, even a 5 per cent infection rate will double or triple the adult death rate. In a middle-income developing country with adult mortality of one per 1,000, the same endemic level of HIV infection will increase prime-age adult mortality five or tenfold.

Given these parameters, how much will the epidemic increase the demand for care? In a country where adults consume one-quarter of health care prior to the AIDS epidemic, HIV prevalence is constant at 5 per cent of adults, the median time to death is ten years and the baseline mortality rate among prime-age adults is 5 per 1,000, the epidemic will cause a 26 per cent increase in the demand for health care at every price. If the prevalence rate is higher, the median time to death shorter, or the baseline adult mortality rate smaller, the percentage increase in demand will be correspondingly greater.

Another important factor that may increase demand is insurance. This may take the form of private insurance, a government-run insurance program, or, more typically, health care financed through general taxation. Because a portion of health care costs is often covered by one or more of these types of insurance, the price paid by the patient is usually a fraction of the cost of providing the care.

Since insurance enables patients to purchase more care than they would otherwise, it increases the demand for care arising from any given level of illness, thus magnifying the price shock of an AIDS epidemic. For example, if the proportion of cost of providing care paid by patients (*i.e.*, the coinsurance rate) is 25 per cent, patients will reduce their utilisation in response to increased cost by only a quarter as much as they would if they had to pay the full increase.

Reduced supply of health care: In addition to increasing the demand for care, the AIDS epidemic will reduce the supply available at a given price, in three ways. The magnitude of these effects, discussed below, will generally be larger in the poorest countries with the largest epidemics. The first and largest effect is the increased cost of maintaining a given level of safety for medical procedures. Even without HIV, hospitals and clinics in poor countries may pose a risk to health.

Because the AIDS epidemic has greatly increased the risk to patients of existing medical procedures, simply maintaining the level of safety that existed before HIV requires additional hygiene and blood screening, both of which increase the cost of care. In middle to high-income countries, where blood screening and sterilisation of injecting equipment are already the norm, the impact of AIDS is confined to the incremental costs of adding an HIV test to existing tests and using rubber gloves and face masks in situations where they were previously not used.

In poor countries, where blood screening and needle sterilisation were lacking before the epidemic, the resources needed to maintain the quality of care in the face of the AIDS epidemic can be substantial. For example, the annual recurrent budget of the Ugandan Blood Transfusion Service, which was established in response to the epidemic and meets the demands of the entire Ugandan national health care system for clean blood, is estimated to be about $1.2 million, including capital and recurrent costs.

This amounts to about 2 per cent of national public health expenditures or about 1 per cent of total national health expenditures. Despite the potentially high costs of blood screening, HIV has greatly increased the justification for a government role in ensuring a safe blood supply. However, there is no convincing rationale for government to subsidize the entire cost of running such a service indefinitely. Blood screening and improved collection procedures will protect blood donors and recipients.

However, since average donors and recipients do not engage in unprotected sex with a large number of partners, a person infected while giving or receiving blood is not likely to pass the infection to many others. Thus, in developing countries where the cost of establishing a safe blood supply is high, blood screening will not be among the more cost-effective approaches to preventing an epidemic based on sexual transmission. To be sure, blood screening and better hygiene will help to prevent the spread of other infectious diseases besides AIDS. Such measures will also reduce the occupational risk of AIDS and other diseases that health care workers face and therefore reduce the amount of additional compensation needed to offset their occupational risk—an issue we discuss below.

A careful accounting of the net cost of protecting patients from HIV by screening blood would need to take into consideration these additional benefits, for which data are lacking. However, it seems likely that even if these benefits are taken into account, the remaining cost of screening blood and improving hygiene to protect patients from HIV/AIDS would substantially increase the unit cost of medical care.

The second factor reducing the supply of medical care at a given price is the increased attrition of health care workers who become infected with HIV. Like all adults, health care workers may become infected with HIV as a result of sexual contact or use of unsterile injecting equipment. They also face an additional risk of becoming infected in the course of their work; however, this risk is generally much smaller than the risk from sexual contact.

Thus whether the AIDS mortality rate among health care workers is higher or lower than among the general population depends mostly on the effects of income, education and social status on sexual behaviour. Two studies of HIV prevalence among health care workers from Africa suggest that doctors and nurses are at least as likely to become infected as other people. If this is true elsewhere, a country with stable 5 per cent HIV prevalence can expect that each year between .5 and 1 per cent of its health care providers will die from AIDS; a country with 30 per cent prevalence would lose 3 to 7 per cent of its health care workers to the epidemic.

This attrition from AIDS deaths may substantially increase the cost of health care. For example, if labour costs are half of total health care costs and training or recruiting a replacement worker requires a one-time expenditure equal to the worker's annual salary, then a 7 per cent increase in attrition will increase total costs in the health sector by 3.5 percent.

The third way in which AIDS reduces the supply of health care is through the additional risk it imposes on health care workers. Even though most HIV-infected health care workers acquire their infection through sexual contact, in a society with a large proportion of HIV positive patients, health care work will be more dangerous than if there were no HIV. Some students who would have become doctors and nurses will therefore choose alternative occupations, unless they are compensated with higher pay for the increased risk.

A recent survey of medical and nursing students in the United States found that AIDS had indeed reduced the attractiveness of specialities in which contact with HIV-positive patients was more likely. This problem is likely to be most severe in hard-hit developing countries, where HIV prevalence is much higher and rubber gloves and other protective equipment are often in short supply.

The magnitude of increased costs of medical staff has not been estimated. Improved precautions in hospitals and clinics may reduce these costs. But because people respond to perceived risk rather than actual risk, such improvements may have little impact on the demand for increased compensation. Thus, it seems clear that health care workers' perception of risk will increase the cost of care. The total impact of these three effects—increased cost of preventing infection in medical facilities, attrition of health care workers due to HIV and additional pay that health care workers demand to compensate them for increased risk—will depend most importantly on HIV prevalence and whether modern blood banks and hygiene were already in place.

In a country that has 5 per cent HIV prevalence among prime-age adults and lacked blood banks and blood screening before the epidemic, a conservative guess is that the cost of providing care of a given quantity and quality will rise by about 10 percent. Scarce care, higher expenditures, taken together the increased demand and reduced supply have two related impacts: first, health care becomes scarcer and thus more expensive. National health care expenditure rises. The size of the increases in health care prices and national health care expenditure depends partly on the price-responsiveness, or "elasticity," of the demand for and supply of care. For most goods, higher prices reduce demand, as consumers switch to substitutes or forgo an intended purchase altogether. This same principle holds true for health care, but the price-responsiveness or elasticity of demand for adult health care is usually small, since there are no close substitutes and people who are sick and who have the ability to pay will often pay whatever is needed to get well.

Higher prices also generally increase supply. Here, too, however, the nature of the health sector affects the supply response. In the very short run, perhaps a month, the supply of care is unlikely to change much. Over the long run, the supply of physicians and inputs to health care can expand as much as necessary.

Over the medium run, five years or so, we would expect the supply of care to respond somewhat to increased demand and the resulting higher price.

A constant 5 per cent seroprevalence rate would eventually increase the demand for care by about one-quarter and the cost of care of a given quality by 10 percent. The increase would be less in a country like India, where only about one-fifth of the cost of care is paid by the government and substantially more in countries like those of Latin America and Eastern Europe, where three-quarters or more of the cost are subsidised.

Although there are significant data problems, the short answer is yes. Measuring the scarcity of medical care through changes in the price of care of given quality is problematical because of the difficulties in measuring quality. This is especially true in developing countries, where a general lack of data is compounded in the health sector by government subsidies and nonprice forms of rationing. In such cases, the effective price of care may rise even though nominal prices remain constant.

Furthermore, because of the lag between infection and death, the time between the attainment of a given HIV prevalence rate and the full impact of that rate on the demand and supply of health care can be 10 to 20 years. For these reasons, we cannot accurately assess changes in scarcity of health care in developing countries by observing changes in nominal price. Nonetheless, we can get some sense of the extent to which HIV/AIDS increases the effective price of health care by considering whether the epidemic makes it more difficult to obtain care. Studies of hospital admissions data strongly suggest that this is the case.

The best evidence that AIDS is making it more difficult for people not infected with the virus to get medical treatment comes from an in-depth study of Kenyatta National Hospital (KNH), the premier teaching hospital in Nairobi, Kenya. The KNH study compared all patients admitted during a sample 22 days in 1988 and 1989 with all patients admitted during a sample 15 days in 1992.

Since the number of HIV-negative people in the hospital's "catchment area" could not have shrunk by this much, this evidence suggests that the AIDS epidemic did in fact result in some HIV-negative patients being dissuaded or barred from admission to the hospital. There are no data on what happened to the HIV-negative patients who were not admitted. But hospital records show that the mortality rates for those who were admitted increased between the two periods, from 14 to 23 per cent. The mortality rate for the HIV-positive patients did not increase and other indicators of the quality of care remained constant.

Thus, the most likely explanation for the increased mortality rate among the HIV-negative patients is that the rationing scheme used to allocate increasingly scarce beds had the effect of changing the mix of HIV-negative patients toward those with more severe illnesses. Whether the rationing was imposed by hospital staff or was a response by prospective patients to their perception of a higher effective price of care, it is likely to have excluded some patients whose lives the hospital could have saved.

Since the HIV-infected make up an increasingly large fraction of the sick people in a severely affected country, it is appropriate that they occupy an increasing share of hospital beds and consume an increasing share of health care resources. The pressure of this increased demand for care will naturally be felt by all citizens, whether or not they are HIV infected.

Scarcer and more expensive care and increased total health expenditure present society with difficult choices. Because a large share of the increased expenditure is typically financed through tax revenues, governments and their constituencies will confront tradeoffs along at least three dimensions:

— treating AIDS versus preventing HIV infection.
— treating AIDS versus treating other illnesses.
— spending for health versus spending for other objectives.

The need to confront these difficult choices can be reduced somewhat if a government is willing and able to increase tax revenues. But few countries will be able to avoid the choices entirely, especially developing countries facing a severe epidemic. Unable to pay for everything, most governments will subsidize some goods and services more than others, thereby disproportionately benefiting certain groups of citizens. As the number of AIDS cases increases, governments are likely to face mounting pressure for two responses that on first consideration seem rational and humane. One is to pay a larger share of health care costs; the other is to provide special subsidies for the treatment of HIV/AIDS. Unfortunately, these responses can have unintended consequences. For reasons discussed below, governments that wish to minimize the impact of HIV on the health sector should try to avoid both courses of action.

However, this does not mean that governments should do nothing to help alleviate the suffering caused by HIV/AIDS. The section concludes with a list of compassionate and affordable measures that governments can and should undertake to mitigate the health sector impact of an HIV/AIDS epidemic.

No increase in the overall subsidy to health care: One obvious and politically appealing response to the HIV/AIDS epidemic is to increase the government share of health care costs and thus the overall subsidy for health care. Such a course of action may be especially attractive early in the epidemic, when few people are sick with AIDS. There is an argument for it on economic grounds as well: it would fill the gap created by the failure of the private market to offer health care insurance in poor countries. However, increasing the subsidy to curative care increases the demand for a limited supply.

As a result, both effective price and total expenditure will rise by a greater proportion than the increased subsidy alone, or the increased demand arising from the epidemic alone, or even the sum of the two, would suggest. As more and more people become sick with AIDS, this effect becomes evident in escalating health care expenditures; in a severe epidemic, the burden on the government budget is likely to become unsustainable. To understand how changes in the level of government subsidies affect the impact of the epidemic on the health care sector, we first look at the extent to which governments already subsidize care.

Then, taking India as an example, we project the impact of an expanding epidemic at the current subsidy level and an increased subsidy level. As we shall see, increasing the overall subsidy to care can greatly exacerbate the impact of the epidemic on the health sector.

India's government health expenditures grow from $3.2 billion in 1991 to $8 billion in 2010. The second line from the bottom shows the increase in government health spending if India's current steep rise in HIV prevalence continues until 2000, then levels off at a stable 5 per cent. This is about the growth in prevalence seen in countries such as Zambia and Botswana, where focused prevention was not implemented early in the epidemic. The result in India would be to increase the government's expenditure on health in the year 2010 by about one-third, from $8 billion to $10.5 billion.

The large expenditure shocks that will result from the AIDS epidemic will create new pressures on health budgets, especially in countries that enter the AIDS epidemic with higher subsidy rates. For example, although Mexico's infection rate was estimated to be only 0.4 per cent in 1994 and it subsidised only 49 per cent of the cost of AIDS treatment, compared with 76 per cent for other sicknesses, AIDS was already consuming 1.2 per cent of its health budget. In contrast, Tanzania has kept the subsidy rate for AIDS treatment down to 28 per cent in line with the subsidy it provides to other illness categories.

As a result, despite a prevalence rate of 5 per cent, more than ten times higher than Mexico's, the AIDS share of total government health care expenditure is only 3.5 per cent, just three times larger in Tanzania than in Mexico. Countries in the nascent or concentrated stages of the epidemic, like India, should carefully consider not only the immediate budgetary consequences of any expanded commitment to fund curative care, but also the multiplication of these consequences that would occur if the AIDS epidemic spreads. A prudent course would be to consider any expansion of government financed health care subsidies or insurance only in conjunction with vigorous prevention programs that enable people most likely to contract and spread HIV to protect themselves and others.

Equal subsidy rates regardless of HIV status: A second common health sector response to the HIV/AIDS epidemic is to offer a different subsidy rate depending on whether or not the person receiving care is infected with HIV. Especially in the countries in the nascent stage of the epidemic, HIV-infected people all too frequently experience discrimination, including restricted access to or higher effective prices for health care.

As the epidemic advances, however, governments are often pressed to provide special subsidies for the treatment of HIV/AIDS. This section points out the government's role in limiting discrimination against the HIV-infected in health care settings and then considers the consequences of preferential subsidies for HIV treatment. AIDS treatment subsidies vary greatly from country to country.

A bias against those with HIV/AIDS can take many forms, ranging from a singling out of AIDS-specific drug therapies for exclusion from public funding, to outright refusal of service. There are many anecdotes about discrimination against the HIV-infected in health care settings. In some hospitals, the HIV-infected were placed in special AIDS wards, which were subsequently shunned by fearful health care workers. In others, the HIV-infected were required to pay extra costs for rubber gloves or a private room.

In still other cases, the HIV-infected have been denied treatment for common illnesses, perhaps because doctors and nurses mistakenly believed that nothing could be done to help a person with HIV/AIDS. Such discrimination is unfair, unprofessional and unethical. Moreover, it displays ignorance of the many ways, discussed above, in which inexpensive treatments for symptoms and opportunistic illnesses can prolong and improve the lives of people with HIV/AIDS.

Government has an important role to play in training medical personnel in order to eradicate all vestiges of discrimination against HIV-infected patients. Yet it is equally unfair and also inefficient, for government to subsidize a higher proportion of the costs of care for patients with HIV than for other patients. Aside from the issue of poverty, there are three ways to justify government subsidies for curative health care: (1) as an incentive for those with an infectious disease to seek a cure and avoid infecting others, (2) as health care insurance with universal coverage and mandatory participation through general taxes, or (3) as government support for a "merit good" or "basic need."

No treatment has yet been shown to reduce the infectivity of sexual contact with an HIV-infected person. AZT treatment of HIV-infected pregnant women has been shown to reduce transmission at birth, but is still too costly an approach to preventing secondary infections in the poorest countries. With the prominent exception of TB, the treatment of which should be subsidized in all countries, most opportunistic illnesses that afflict the HIV infected are infectious only to other equally sick HIV-infected people. Thus the argument for treating the diseases on the grounds that they are infectious is weak. If government subsidy is considered as an insurance payment, efficiency criteria argue for a higher coinsurance (*i.e.*, lower subsidy) rate for any condition in which the patient is likely to be highly price-responsive.

The drugs and medical services to treat AIDS can amount to a great deal of money, although some of the most expensive of these treatments purchase the patient little additional life span and decrease, rather than improve, the quality of life. Thus on efficiency grounds, where the objective is to limit the responsiveness of expenditure to insurance, AIDS patients should face somewhat lower subsidies, not higher ones. The final possibility, that AIDS treatment is a basic need, is difficult to justify in poor countries where the opportunity cost of treating one adult for AIDS may be measles vaccines for 100 to 200 children or, ten student-years of primary school. Thus none of these economic arguments justifies higher subsidy rates for AIDS.

What policy recommendations can be drawn from these two observations? The prudent, efficient and equitable course is to place the financing of health care for HIV/AIDS on the same footing as other diseases. The treatment of particularly infectious illnesses striking HIV infected people, including TB and STDs, should be subsidised relatively generously because of the secondary infections treatment will prevent. Other health care problems of the HIV-infected should be subsidised at the same rate that applies to other adult health problems that are equally infectious.

Affordable, humane responses to the epidemic: We have argued that governments should avoid two types of health care responses to the epidemic: increasing the overall subsidy to all types of treatment and providing disproportionately large subsidies to treatment of HIV/AIDS. There are nonetheless several ways in which governments can intervene to mitigate the health impact of HIV/AIDS on infected individuals and their families and on the overall health sector. Each of these interventions is justified on public economic grounds, either because it has large positive externalities, or because it improves the efficiency or the equity of the health care market in other ways.

— Provide information about the efficacy of treatments. Because people with HIV/AIDS are often desperate for treatment and cannot easily research what works, they are especially vulnerable to quackery. Governments can serve the interests of everyone by promptly investigating unproven treatments and providing credible information about their validity.

— Subsidise the treatment of infectious opportunistic illnesses and STDs. Subsidised treatment is especially appropriate for tuberculosis, one of the most common opportunistic illnesses to infect AIDS patients, since curing a single case can avert many secondary infections. Treatment of gonorrhoea, syphilis and the other classic STDs should be subsidised, not only because they are highly contagious, but also because they exacerbate HIV transmission. Whether a subsidy to antiretroviral treatment of HIV itself is justifiable as a way to prevent secondary HIV infections will depend on the efficacy of the treatment and on its cost relative to the cost of other HIV prevention measures.

— Subsidise the start-up costs for blood safety and AIDS care. The AIDS epidemic has increased the willingness of individuals to pay for certain types of services, such as screening of blood for transfusions and care for the terminally ill. Where these services are lacking, government help with the start-up costs is justified. Thus, governments in poor countries should establish blood banks but should not indefinitely provide free blood. Similarly, government should help establish AIDS treatment facilities, especially community-based home care programs, but should not permanently subsidise the care they provide.

— Provide special assistance to the most poor. Countries already make special provision for medical care to the poor. As the AIDS epidemic increases the demand for care, governments may wish to focus such assistance even more on those who can least afford it. Sliding fee scales and other measures to make care available to the poor should apply to people with HIV/AIDS just as they do to people with other illnesses.

It is sometimes said that "AIDS is a disease of poverty." In what sense might this be true—or false? First, are the poor more likely to become infected with HIV than others? Second, what proportion of people infected with HIV are poor? Answers to these questions are important, for they will influence both the focusing of prevention measures and attempts to mitigate the impact of the AIDS infections that do occur.

HIV infects the rich and the poor: In developing countries, the relationship between income and HIV infection rates has been best documented in eastern and central Africa. Whether the patterns observed in this part of Africa will also emerge elsewhere remains to be seen.

Early in the epidemic in sub-Saharan Africa men and women who travel more and men who had higher incomes, were more likely than others to contract the virus. There are reasons to believe that this may hold true elsewhere. Studies show that sex is similar to other pleasurable pastimes.

This, combined with the fact that HIV unlike other STDs, cannot be readily cured, has made HIV unique among widely prevalent infectious diseases in striking rich people in the same proportion, or larger proportions, than it strikes the poor. That HIV infects the rich as well as the poor is important to keep in mind when considering which households need help the most.

Recent studies in developed countries have shown AIDS incidence to be highest among the very poor perhaps because the literate and wealthy have access to AIDS-related information. If these trends are replicated worldwide, AIDS will become like other infectious diseases, in that the poor will be more likely, to become infected than the un-poor. Ultimately, AIDS may become most prevalent in the poorest urban slums of developing countries.

Already, most people with HIV/AIDS are poor. Although lack of data makes it impossible to calculate the precise proportions of poor and un-poor who are infected, knowledge of income levels and infection rates across countries suggests that many more poor people are infected than nonpoor people.

If we assume that one of government's main responsibilities is to make it possible for people to escape from poverty, these findings lead us to new questions. What is the impact on a poor household when the mother, father, or another prime-age adult who is a member of the household dies from AIDS? How do poor households cope with AIDS deaths?

How households cope with the impact of adult death: The economic shock of a prime-age adult death would have been larger and more persistent, except that households use a variety of strategies to cope. Before the AIDS epidemic, prime-age adult deaths were much less common, so these mechanisms were used mostly to cope with other shocks. As a result, early assessments of the household impact of AIDS tended to overlook household coping and assume that AIDS would be catastrophic not only for the infected individual but also for the entire household.

Press accounts that presented devastated households as typical contributed to the widespread belief that most AIDS affected households in developing countries would collapse. To be sure, some households are destroyed by AIDS; this is especially true if both parents become ill or die while their children are still very young. However, such instances may be less typical than is generally assumed because of the typically long lag between HIV infection and death.

Understanding the variety of household coping mechanisms and how these will affect different groups of households is important. The mix of responses attempted by a specific household in response to a prime-age adult death depends on countless factors, some of which will vary across countries and communities.

Since the available data on household impact comes mostly from Sub-Saharan Africa, the following discussion unavoidably reflects this bias. Policymakers in all countries faced with the possibility of a generalised epidemic will want to assess the extent to which these responses are evident in their own country. To varying degrees, however, three coping mechanisms observed in Africa—altering household composition, drawing down savings or selling assets and utilising assistance from other households—are all likely to be attempted whenever households confront the tragedy of a prime-age adult death.

Altering household composition. Households everywhere fulfil economic as well as social functions. In rural areas of developing countries, households are often the main production unit for subsistence farming and, in some instances, for cash crop farming as well. In such a situation, the economic shock of the death of a prime-age adult can be cushioned to some degree by altering household composition. Examples of such changes could include sending one or more dependent children to live with relatives, or inviting an unmarried aunt or uncle to join the household in exchange for assistance with farming and household tasks.

Results from three of the four available household surveys—two from Africa and one from Chiang Mai, Thailand—show that the degree to which household composition is used to cushion the shock of the death varies according to the size and flexibility of local household structure. Among the 759 households in the Kagera, Tanzania study interviewed once every six months for two years, 130 household members of all ages died, but roughly nine times as many people left the households alive over the same period and seven times as many joined the households. In addition, about 200 children were born to household members.

During the six months between any two interviews, economically active adults left or joined about one-fifth of the households that did not have an adult death and about 40 per cent of the households that did suffer a death. Since most households that suffered a death added at least one member, the average size of these households declined by less than one, from 6.4 to 5.7 members—so that the average household size after a death was the same as in households that did not suffer a death. Similarly, the dependency ratio rose only slightly in households with an adult death, from

1.2 to 1.4, slightly less than the 1.5 dependency ratio in households without an adult death. A striking fact is that household size and dependency ratios changed very little, even though Kagera has high adult mortality from AIDS. The same phenomenon was observed in the survey in Rakai, Uganda, which, like Kagera, has a severe AIDS epidemic: 15 per cent or more of adults in roadside communities are infected with HIV. This suggests that, even in a generalised AIDS epidemic, most African households that suffer an AIDS death will be able to adjust household size and dependency ratios in ways that make them similar to households that did not suffer a death.

There are two points of similarity between the household composition responses to death in the Kagera and Chiang Mai studies. First, the Chiang Mai households with deaths, like their Kagera counterparts, suffered an increased dependency ratio due to the deaths. Because of the smaller number of adults in the Thai households, the dependency ratio there almost doubled after the death.

Second, in both countries households with a death were twice as likely to experience membership change as the households without deaths. However, the proportion of households that experienced a membership change and the rates of turnover were only about one-quarter as large in Chiang Mai as in Kagera.

Households may respond opportunistically by moving people into a household that is benefiting from an assistance program. The evidence here suggests that, even if this turns out to be a problem in Africa, it is much less likely to be an issue in places like Chiang Mai where households are much smaller and apparently less able or willing to adjust their membership in response to outside stimuli.

Dissavings and the sale of assets: Drawing down savings and selling assets is an obvious potential mechanism for coping with prime-age adult death. Because assets may have been accumulated as part of a strategy to cushion unanticipated shocks, drawing upon them is one of the least painful ways of coping, much less painful than reducing food consumption, for example. Evidence from Kagera,

Rakai and Chiang Mai suggests that households do draw down savings or liquidate assets in response to a prime-age adult death.

The surveys in Kagera and Rakai both asked respondents about their ownership of three types of durable goods: a car or truck, a bicycle and a radio. Less than 2 per cent of the households owned a car or lorry and changes in ownership did not show any clear pattern in relation to whether households suffered an adult death. However, ownership of bicycles and radios, which is much more widespread, did reveal a pattern.

In both surveys, radio ownership increased among households that had no death and decreased among households that had a death. A similar pattern can be seen for bicycle ownership in Rakai, although not in Kagera. Thus the evidence from Rakai, partially supported by the Kagera data, suggests that some households that suffer an adult death may be selling durable goods as part of their coping strategy. The alternative is that these goods may have belonged to the deceased and been willed to someone outside the household. Even in this instance, however, the loss of the asset may help with coping efforts, if the recipient feels an increased obligation to assist the bereaved.

Additional evidence of households drawing down savings to cope with an adult death can be seen in Kagera data on membership in traditional rotating savings and credit associations (ROSCAs). In wave 1 of the survey, 51 per cent of the 80 households that would experience an adult death during the eighteen-month survey period were members of a ROSCA; by the end of the survey, participation had dropped to 36 percent. Among households that did not experience a death during the survey period, ROSCA participation varied less, from 41 per cent in wave 1 to 36 per cent in wave 4.

Although the Chiang Mai survey does not permit comparisons of financial variables over time between households that experienced a death and those that did not, fully 41 per cent of households with a death report having sold land, 57 per cent report some dissavings and 24 per cent report borrowing from a cooperative or revolving fund (*i.e.*, a ROSCA) to finance the adjustment to the death. Perhaps it is the greater wealth of the Thai households that permitted them to cushion the shock in these ways, rather than through readjustment of household composition.

Assistance from other households: For all households confronted with an adult death, help from relatives and neighbours is a potentially important supplement to the household's own efforts. Policymakers considering how to best use the limited resources for mitigating the household impact will want to avoid displacing such private transfers. To do so, they will need information about assistance from households in the specific communities concerned. The discussion that follows is not intended to substitute for this information, but only to suggest the types and possible relative magnitude of such responses. An important feature of the social organisation of Kagera households and indeed of most African communities, is interdependence in time of need.

In Kagera, both bereaved and nonbereaved households were very likely to receive cash or in-kind assistance from other households. (About three-quarters of the nonbereaved households received such assistance, compared with 80 to 90 per cent of the households that suffered a death.) But among households that received private transfers after a death, the median amount received during the half-year of the death ($53) was more than twice that received during the year before the death, as well as twice that received by households that did not suffer a death. New organisations established to help cope with the costs of AIDS death may be one explanation for this large difference. Focus group interviews in 20 of the sample villages found that besides traditional savings and mutual assistance associations, such as ROSCAs, residents of many villages had launched associations specifically to help families affected by an AIDS death. Most of these associations were launched and operated by women; many have regular meetings at which members make contributions in cash or in kind.

Assistance from government and NGOs: Regarding assistance from government and NGOs, two types of questions must be asked. First, which families receive such assistance and how much do they receive? Second, how much does it cost to provide this assistance? Cost considerations did not figure in our discussion of private assistance, since only private resources are involved. But governments and NGOs use public resources, whether generated by taxes or by voluntary contributions.

Accordingly, we should ask whether these funds are used in the most effective way possible. In this discussion, assistance from government and NGOs is referred to as program transfers or formal assistance, to distinguish it from the private and informal assistance provided by households and village associations.

According to the Kagera survey, program transfers reached fewer households and provided a smaller amount of assistance than private transfers. In the last wave of the survey, one-fifth of the households that had not had an adult death in the past eighteen months had received assistance from an organisation in the past six months; almost two-fifths of the households that had experienced a death received such assistance. The median value of program assistance received was small relative to total household expenditure and to the amounts of private assistance received.

But while, on average, households that had experienced a death received larger amounts of assistance, this was not always the case. Nor were program transfers always small relative to annual income. In one village, 50 per cent of the households, including some that had never reported a death, received more than $110 in program transfers during the six months before wave 4.

To analyse the relative costs of various types of programs for assisting households affected by AIDS and other causes of adult death, the survey collected data from one governmental and eleven nongovernmental organisations operating in the Kagera Region.

In considering the implied cost comparisons, it is important to remember that the services provided may be very different; for example, home care focuses on the sick household member, while educational support helps dependent children, who may not be sick, to attend school. Furthermore, even the programs averaged in a single category often contain disparate program elements and vary in quality.

There can be very large differences in the cost per beneficiary of different types of programs. A particularly telling comparison is between the cost of supporting a child in a foster home, estimated at $107 per year and the cost of supporting a child in an orphanage, which averages $1,063, or ten times larger. For children who cannot be placed in a foster home, it may be necessary to consider the alternative of an orphanage. However, policymakers and NGO providers should keep in mind that every child sent to an orphanage will consume the resources that could have been used to support ten children in foster homes.

The economic impact of AIDS is larger in poor households: Households that experience an adult death draw on their assets to cushion the shock of this catastrophe. It follows that households with lower levels of assets can be expected to have more difficulty coping with the death than households with more assets.

Impact on food consumption: The greater impact of a prime-age adult death on poorer households appears most starkly in changes in food expenditure and food consumption. For the better-off households, both measures of food intake increased. The picture is quite different for the poorest 50 per cent of the households: food expenditure, which was already lower in these households than in the others, dropped by nearly a third. The resulting drop in per capita food consumption was cushioned by an increase in the consumption of home-produced food.

Even so, per capita consumption in the poorer households fell by 15 percent. Even if these households eventually return almost to the pre-death level of per capita food consumption, as did the Ivoirian households, lack of adequate nutrition for a year or more can have a profound effect on the development of children.

Impact on child nutrition: Childhood malnutrition is potentially one of the most severe and lasting consequences of a prime-age adult death. The death of a parent or other adult may lower the nutritional status of surviving children by reducing household income and food expenditure and by reducing adult attention to childrearing. Because childhood malnutrition can impede intellectual development and thus reduce a person's long-run productivity, improving childhood nutrition has long been an important development goal. Policymakers seeking to mitigate the impact of the AIDS epidemic will therefore be particularly concerned about minimising the impact of the increasing number of prime-age adult deaths on childhood nutrition. The impact of adult death on childhood nutrition is likely to vary according to many factors, not least of which is the nutritional status of children in the overall population. Little information is available on how adult death affects child nutrition. Moreover, the impact is likely to differ across countries and communities.

Programs that provide food directly to malnourished children and to orphans, rather than to households that include orphans, may avoid the problem of households fostering children primarily to obtain benefits intended for the orphans. While creating an incentive for households to foster children may be desirable in a severe AIDS epidemic, too large an incentive can increase the number of children shifted between households, to the detriment of their welfare. A better approach may be to include children in households where a death is anticipated in community-based nutrition monitoring and feeding programs on the model of the UNICEF-sponsored "village feeding posts."

Finally, including orphans in a program designed to address malnutrition more broadly is more equitable than focusing assistance on AIDS orphans alone. This is particularly true in very poor countries, where an alarmingly high proportion of all children are malnourished. In Kagera, for example, even in households that are less poor and have both parents alive, nearly one-third of children are stunted. In such a situation, providing assistance only to AIDS orphans would neglect a large number of children who are also very needy.

Impact on child schooling: Besides increasing childhood malnutrition, a prime-age adult death in a household is likely to reduce school enrolment. This lack of schooling, perhaps exacerbated by inadequate nutrition, will make it particularly difficult for child survivors of a prime-age adult death to escape poverty. The effects of a prime-age death that could decrease enrolment among children in the household include:

— reducing the ability of families to pay for schooling.

— raising the demand for children's labour.

— reducing the expected return to adults of investments in children's schooling.

Children may also be withdrawn from school to work outside the home, help with chores and farming, or care for an ailing family member. In addition, where prime-age adult mortality is high, parents may be less willing to invest in their children's schooling, either because they fear that the children will not live long enough to realise the higher earnings schooling promises, or because the parents themselves do not expect to live long enough to benefit from their children's future earnings.

Similarly, relatives who take in an orphan may be less willing than the parents would have been to invest in the child's schooling. For all these reasons, children who have lost one or both parents are likely to have lower enrolment rates than those whose parents are alive.

Data from the Demographic and Health Surveys on enrolment and orphanhood in nine countries generally support this premise. Orphans have significantly lower enrolment rates in every area except Uganda and Zimbabwe; differences in enrolment rates of orphans and nonorphans are greatest in the five sets of bars on the left. But while the data support the view that orphans are less likely to attend school than other children, they also clearly demonstrate that in most of these countries a very large proportion of children who are not orphans are also not attending school.

POVERTY POLICY IN A SEVERE AIDS EPIDEMIC

Although it already infects more poor people than rich people and will probably eventually infect a higher proportion of the poor, many HIV infections continue to occur among the nonpoor. The short-term impact of a prime-age adult death is higher for AIDS than for other causes of death, primarily because of the long illness that often precedes an AIDS death. However, because other costs are incurred in all cases of adult death, the overall difference in the short-term impact of AIDS deaths and other deaths is not large.

Rather than being destroyed by AIDS, households use a variety of mechanisms to cushion the short-term impact of an AIDS or other prime-age adult death. We have seen that these coping mechanisms are much less effective in poor households, where more of the coping is at the expense of children's school enrolment and nutritional status.

Because the problems are relatively new and there are very few comparable data across countries, or indeed even across regions within a country, we have relied heavily on a single survey in Kagera, Tanzania, with additional observations from three other recent surveys in other countries. As experience with the AIDS epidemic increases and additional data become available, our understanding will certainly improve and some of the observations here will be challenged.

In poor developing regions, many households that have not been affected by AIDS are likely to be very poor. Among the Kagera households that had not experienced an adult death, one-third of the children under 5 were stunted. Similarly, even in households where both parents were alive, 50 per cent of the children under 11 were not enrolled in school.

While the households affected by AIDS are not necessarily poor, the poor households that are affected are much less able to cope than the non poor households. Less-poor households in Kagera actually experienced an increase in consumption per capita after the death, while the poorest households experienced a sharp reduction in consumption, especially food consumption, as a result of the death. While the increased consumption in the nonpoor households will not necessarily be observed in other locales, it is reasonable to assume that nonpoor households faced with an adult death will be much better placed to smooth consumption than poor households.

Even households that lack access to formal credit and insurance markets nonetheless use a variety of measures to cope with AIDS deaths and other misfortunes. Thus, even if the shock from an AIDS death is larger than that from other misfortunes and poor households are more vulnerable to the shock than nonpoor households, governments seeking to mitigate the impact of AIDS on poverty must ask themselves whether it is possible to design and implement, either directly or through NGOs, assistance programs that are more efficient and equitable than the informal coping strategies already in place.

These broad findings can be further distilled into three general recommendations for policymakers:

— Not all households experiencing an AIDS death need assistance.

— If survivor assistance is to be offered, it should be targeted to all very poor households that suffer a prime-age adult death, regardless of whether the death was due to AIDS.

— Assistance will do the most good immediately before and after the adult death, during the period when per capita food consumption has fallen but not yet recovered. It need not be permanent.

In addition to these three points, there is potentially important synergy between AIDS mitigation and antipoverty programs. For example, the finding that poor households are more vulnerable to the impact of an AIDS death implies that general antipoverty policies can also be AIDS mitigation policies. If general antipoverty policies are effective in reducing the number of poor households, then AIDS deaths will occur in stronger households that can cope at smaller, cost to the survivors.

Similarly, an adult death depresses per capita food consumption in the poorest households by 15 per cent implies that AIDS deaths that occur in poor households exacerbate poverty. Thus, when AIDS mitigation policies are targeted to households that were poor before the AIDS death, they are likely to prevent the affected household from slipping further into misery as a result of the death. In this case, AIDS mitigation policies could be effective at limiting the depth, if not the extent, of poverty.

Antipoverty programs and mitigation programs be integrated. When an antipoverty program is designed for a community with low living standards, consideration should be given to including components that specifically address the needs of the poorest households hit by AIDS deaths.

For example, suppose the antipoverty program in a specific AIDS-affected community consists of a labour-intensive public works program. Components that would generate such synergy might include:

- home-based or hostel-based care for the terminally ill to enable healthy adults who would otherwise have provided this care to take advantage of the jobs.
- day-care centers or "feeding posts" to enable single parents to take the jobs.

When a mitigation program is established, locating it close to and combining it with a conventional antipoverty program will improve its effectiveness. In an area severely affected by an AIDS epidemic, implementing either program in isolation from the other sacrifices an opportunity for effective development policy.

Although the specifics of the impacts on health and poverty differ, the analysis leads to broadly similar conclusions in both areas. Special government assistance for people infected with HIV/AIDS and their survivors must be weighed carefully against the many other pressing needs that governments face. Well-intentioned government efforts to assist individuals with HIV/AIDS and their families may divert resources from other families that have not been afflicted by HIV/AIDS but are nonetheless suffering from illness, poverty, or both. In particular, HIV-infected patients should be responsible for the same portion of the cost of their care as other patients with similar income and likelihood of infecting others.

Because of HIV's long incubation period, governments may initially underestimate the cost of programs to provide special assistance to those affected by HIV/AIDS. As the number of people who get sick and die from the disease increases, these programs will absorb a growing share of resources that could have been used to address other problems. Because AIDS may divert resources from other pressing problems and commit governments to expenditures from which it will later be politically difficult to withdraw, policymakers in developing countries should be wary of programs that provide special assistance to people with HIV and their families solely on the basis of an HIV diagnosis.

HIV would be a serious but manageable health challenge, perhaps not unlike cancer or other difficult-to-treat diseases, rather than a global epidemic. Unfortunately, national and international efforts to fight AIDS are far from optimal. Fifteen years into the epidemic, many developing country governments still lack adequate surveillance systems and have yet to enable a large enough share of those who are most likely to contract and spread HIV to protect themselves and others. Moreover, many countries also lack the society- wide policies to support such prevention interventions.

Despite the willingness of non-profit private groups to contribute to the fight against AIDS, some governments have difficulty providing the right mix of support and supervision. Donor governments and multilateral organisations, which provide much of the financing for national AIDS programs, have not always encouraged recipient governments to set and address appropriate priorities and they have invested too little in international public goods: knowledge and technology for fighting the epidemic in developing countries.

Why has the national and international policy response to the AIDS epidemic not been more satisfactory? Much of the explanation involves an understandable lack of knowledge. AIDS is a relatively recent challenge. Faced with a potential emergency, governments, donors and multilateral organisations responded as best they knew how use the information that available. As knowledge about the epidemic and ways to combat it increases, public responses are likely to improve. Like all public policies, however, AIDS policy is not made in a vacuum. Indeed, because the spread of HIV involves private behaviour that many people deplore—frequent changes in sexual partners and the injection of addictive drugs—governments that adopt programs to reduce the riskiness of these activities may be accused by their constituents of facilitating socially deviant or immoral behaviour.

Thus HIV/AIDS policy may be subject to strong political pressures, some of which work against the policies most likely to contain the epidemic. In considering these issues, we looks beyond the national policies to consider how the main actors in the AIDS policy arena can work together to more effectively confront the epidemic.

Government, donors and NGOs

Mostly government bear the responsibility for protecting their citizens from the spread of the HIV epidemic and of mitigating its worst effects once it has spread. But they are not alone in the effort. Bilateral and multilateral donors have provided both leadership and major funding for national AIDS prevention programs, especially in the poorer developing countries. And both local and international nongovernmental organisations have stepped forward to help against the epidemic, sometimes prodding reluctant governments into action. The challenge for national governments is to define their role in the struggle against the epidemic, not in isolation from or in passive response to the other actors, but in active collaboration with them.

Only the government can claim to represent and act on behalf of the national population. Among the three types of actors, it has the unique ability to authorize implementation of an intervention by a donor or NGO. However, a donor cannot be commanded to finance or implement a program in which it has little interest. NGOs, too, have preferences and technical strengths or weaknesses. Thus the government cannot simply assign tasks to itself and the other actors. Instead it must learn the preferences and judge the comparative advantages of donors and NGOs. If there are important tasks that public economics considerations assign to the public sector, but that donors and NGOs either cannot or will not perform, then the government must undertake them directly or subcontract them. What roles have the three sets of actors played in the struggle against the AIDS epidemic? How can cooperation be improved to make the most of the strengths of each?

Although the data on financing are incomplete and imprecise, they present a coherent picture of the relative roles of national governments and donors in developing countries: donors have assumed the major financing burden in the poorest developing countries and bilateral donors show a preference for countries suffering from generalised epidemics.

Since the available cross-country data speak only to financing, the analysis of the NGOs' role in implementation is based on examples. Although no generalisation regarding roles will apply to every country, the analysis suggests that many national governments and NGOs should assume a somewhat larger share of the funding of prevention activities, leaving donors to focus on the international public goods discussed in the next section. Furthermore, anecdotal evidence supports the claim that the donors frequently work at cross-purposes at the country level. Efforts would be more effective if donors would improve their coordination with one another and with national authorities without slowing the speed with which they deliver assistance.

The total amount of donor funding for AIDS was estimated at approximately $300 million in 1996. The largest contributor of new funds in that year was the United States ($117 million); the European Union ($55 million) and Japan ($40 million) provided the next largest amounts of grant funding and the World Bank provided approximately $45 million in new loan commitments that year, most of which was at concessional rates. This seemingly large amount of money is, however, only about 6 per cent of total donor health assistance to developing countries.

Nevertheless, since AIDS expenditures represent a substantial fraction of total public spending on health in some developing countries, observers have asked whether too large a proportion of health resources is devoted to AIDS in these countries relative to other health problems.

The WHO Global Programme on AIDS, predecessor of UNAIDS, collected data on donor, national and NGO funding of AIDS programs in participating countries for the period 1991-93. While this database is imperfect and under-represents funding from national and NGO sources, it provides the only detailed view of AIDS funding for a significant number of developing countries.

Average annual 1991-93 spending on AIDS by donors recorded by the GPA funding database exceeded 10 per cent of 1990 public health spending in only seven countries: Uganda (59%), Tanzania (36%) Zambia (27%), Malawi (16%), Central African Republic (13%), Guinea (11%) and Rwanda (11). In these seven countries, all of which are in Africa and have some of the most serious AIDS epidemics in the world, international AIDS spending is large enough to overshadow all other prevention programs operated by the ministries of health.

International spending was greater than 1 per cent of the public health budget in 32 additional countries, including the non-African countries of Haiti (7 percent), Vietnam (3 percent), Thailand (3 percent), Lao PDR (3 percent), Bolivia (3 percent), Bangladesh (2 percent), Sri Lanka (2 percent), Pakistan 0.4 percent), Honduras (1.1 percent) and Chile (1.01 percent).

Countries with large ratios of donor-funded AIDS spending to total national health spending are the exception rather than the rule. The average country in fact received a little less than 2 per cent of its 1990 health budget for AIDS. Even in low-income countries with generalised epidemics, the average percentage of the national health budget received for AIDS was only 8.5 percent. The average percentage of the health budget received from donors for AIDS declines from 3.2 per cent among the low-income countries to one-tenth of a per cent among the upper-middle-income countries.

This is due to higher total public health spending in the higher-income countries, as well as to lower donor allocations to these countries. Looking across stages of the epidemic, we see that donor funding as an average percentage of national health spending rose consistently from one-third of a per cent in the nascent countries to nearly 8 per cent in the countries with generalised epidemics. However, even the higher figure does not threaten to overwhelm ministries or to overshadow other public health programs in the average recipient country.

If donor-funded AIDS spending is occasionally large compared with the national health budget, national AIDS program spending never exceeds 10 per cent of total national health spending and only rarely exceeds 1 percent, as judged from the survey of national program spending conducted for AIDS.

Although donor allocations for AIDS are not large enough to overwhelm the domestic health care system in most developing countries, these allocations are remarkably large relative to national spending on the same problem and probably in comparison with current international spending on any other disease. Perhaps only the international campaign to eradicate smallpox in the 1970s benefited from such a large preponderance of donor funds. But the amount of both types of funding varies a great deal from one country to the next. The next section seeks to explain this variation.

The severity of the epidemic and the availability of resources should be the two primary determinants of the extent of HIV/AIDS interventions in a developing country. Furthermore, the absolute size of a country's population will affect the scale of activities and therefore of expenditure. How does spending vary across countries by infection rate, GDP per capita and population size? To avoid double-counting the HIV infected, the analysis below breaks the population into two components, the number infected and the number not infected. It then examines their separate influence and that of GDP per capita, on aggregate levels of national and international AIDS expenditures in a country. More than 60 per cent of the cross-country pattern of domestically financed AIDS expenditures can be explained by these three variables. The analysis focuses on the number of people infected and on GDP per capita to see how these two variables affect national and international allocations for confronting AIDS.

It is not surprising that national and international decisionmakers respond to the severity of the AIDS epidemic. It is reasonable for governments to respond to evidence of HIV infection with increased funding for both prevention and curative programs. National governments that view the epidemic with urgency might be expected to respond more strongly to HIV infections than would international donors, not less so. One possible explanation for the weakness of the national governments' spending response to the epidemic might be the availability of international donor funding. If this were true, one would expect that some of the variation in national expenditure, after controlling for HIV infections and the other variables, could be explained by the receipt of donor funds.

There is no statistically significant correlation between national and donor funding in a country. Moreover, this is true even if we correct for the influence on national expenditure of GDP per capita, the number infected with HIV and the number not infected. Although some individual governments undoubtedly made their decisions on national funding levels based on what they were receiving from outside, this evidence suggests that this is not the case for the average country.

Turning to GDP per capita, we see in the left-hand panel that national spending is extremely responsive to national income of two countries of the same size and the same number of HIV-infected people, the one that is 10 per cent poorer spends about 12 per cent less on managing its AIDS epidemic. And the fit to that relationship is quite good. This striking sensitivity to income level could be explained as the rational response by decisionmakers who have full information about the danger of AIDS and the role of the public sector in confronting it but are not convinced that government intervention can slow the epidemic and are acutely aware of the many other demands on extremely scarce public resources.

Under this interpretation, national decisionmakers view AIDS expenditures as a luxury, affordable only at higher income levels. Alternatively, it could be that decisionmakers in lower-income countries have less complete information about AIDS than those in other countries and perhaps are handicapped to a greater degree by conservative constituencies. Either of these interpretations suggests that donor assistance is acutely needed in the lowest-income countries to enable significant national activity against AIDS. But the latter interpretation, further argues that low-income countries should strive to increase their national effort against AIDS in order to ensure that people most likely to contract and spread HIV are able to protect themselves and others.

Thus many factors besides population size, epidemic severity and GNP per capita influence international assistance to a country's AIDS program. While donors must and should take many other considerations into account, this evidence suggests that donors should give greater consideration to per capita income than they did from 1991 to 1993 when determining how to allocate resources to confront AIDS across countries, so that low-income countries with severe epidemics would be sure to receive the resources needed for the essential core functions of an AIDS program.

Multilateral funding and stage of epidemic

While bilaterals allocated the lion's share of their AIDS assistance ($316 million, or 63 percent) to countries in the generalised stage of the epidemic, multilaterals allocated the bulk of their assistance ($379 million, or 62 percent) to countries in the concentrated stage of the epidemic. International NGOs accounted for only a small portion of total funding reported in the database; the 16.4 million they provided was about equally split between countries with concentrated epidemics and countries with generalised epidemics.

This discrepancy between the funding patterns of bilaterals and multilaterals may have been only temporary and was perhaps partly due to two large World Bank loans made to India and Brazil during this period, both of which have concentrated epidemics. However, the pattern casts doubt on the frequent assertion that countries with advanced epidemics will encounter donor "fatigue" from bilateral donors and be forced to turn to multilaterals as the funders of last resort.

The observed pattern suggests instead that the bilaterals are particularly concerned about countries where the caseload is highest. Such behaviour is consistent with two views of the motives of bilaterals. Perhaps they are altruistically responding to the suffering of countries with generalised epidemics. Or perhaps they view their self-interest as jeopardised most acutely by countries where there are large numbers of infected people. Whatever their motive, the bilateral focus on countries with generalised epidemics has left multilaterals to fund countries at the nascent and concentrated stages. The outcome of this division of responsibility is that countries where the epidemic is nascent or concentrated pay higher costs for their external AIDS funding than those where it is generalised, but it does ensure that funds are available for all countries. It also permits donor governments to focus their resources on hard-hit countries where their constituencies are likely to most support spending.

Achieving the most cost-effective response to the HIV/AIDS epidemic requires cooperation between governments and NGOs, both non-profit and for-profit. But working with NGOs can be costly for governments. Governments need to develop and apply guidelines and procedures to assure that the collaborative relationship operates with minimal friction and maximum effect. Many of the highest-priority interventions require delivering highly differentiated services to small distinctive groups of clients, such as sex workers or poor AIDS-affected households.

Effective service delivery requires the ability to learn from and respond quickly to, the changing needs of a specific subpopulation. Because the needs of one client group are different from those of the next, unit costs are likely to rise rather than fall when the same organisation attempts to deliver to multiple groups. In this situation, service delivery costs less if undertaken by many small entities rather than by one large one, such as a government agency.

When a highly differentiated service has the attributes of a public good, local communities often spontaneously create a nonprofit, grass roots NGO to deliver them, endowing it with finances and volunteer labour. However, in developing countries many local communities lack the internal organisation or resources to create their own NGOs and few have sufficient incentives or resources to subsidize services whose benefits extend beyond their boundaries. Thus, governments cannot expect spontaneously created NGOs to tackle the epidemic alone. NGOs need the public mandate, technical information, financing and sector coordination that governments can provide, while governments need NGOs for their diversity, flexibility, potential cost-effectiveness and credibility with marginalised people. By working together, NGOs and governments can be a formidable force in the struggle against HIV/AIDS.

Once government has identified an AIDS-related service that is undersupplied by the private market, it must ask the question whether it is possible to (1) precisely specify in a written contract the quantity and quality of the service to be provided and (2) monitor the contract for compliance.

It might be difficult to specify a complete contract either because the quality of the service depends on subjective aspects of its delivery (for example, the kindness and solicitude of an individual delivering home-based care), or because even the physical aspects of service delivery are difficult to measure (for example, whether the condoms reportedly sold to sex workers really went to them or were instead sold to pharmacies catering to the middle class).

Monitoring might be difficult for technical reasons (for example, the presence of a government representative in the room to watch an NGO member educate prisoners or sex workers might destroy the rapport between educator and clients), or a government might simply not have sufficient trained and motivated personnel to monitor a large number of NGO contracts. When the contract can be specified accurately and monitored for compliance, the government can choose among all the available NGO candidates, including both for-profit and nonprofit firms, depending only on their technical qualifications for the task at hand.

In such circumstances the winning candidate will often be a for-profit firm with no direct ties to any client constituency, because they typically have the capability to mobilise the best expertise in the country, to produce outputs to international standards of excellence, to follow government or donor guidelines regarding records and accounts, to minimize costs and to raise capital for expansion as needed to fulfil the contract. However, since it typically has no other constituency to satisfy, a for-profit firm will reduce its costs, not only by eliminating waste, but also by reducing the quantity or quality of any unmonitored dimension of service.

When the contract for a highly differentiated service is difficult to specify or monitor, there is a strong argument for the government to favour an NGO that has its own constituency with a stake in the quality of the service. In contrast to the for-profit firm, which might divert resources in order to maximize profits, the nonprofit NGO has the incentive to divert resources toward the other services it provides or toward advocacy. Thus, governments considering delegation to an NGO as a solution to their inability to completely monitor performance must consider the conformity of the NGOs' overall objectives with the public interest.

Different types of nonprofit NGOs have different overall objectives. Broad-based public charities have large constituencies drawn from the general public and are therefore likely to have objectives in broad conformity with the general public interest. However, such broad-based public charities are likely to be less credible with the client groups than an organisation composed of members of that group. Therefore, in selecting an NGO for a specific contract, governments may face a tradeoff between the degree to which the organisation's objectives conform to those of the general public and the organisation's effectiveness in working with the specific client group.

There are four stylised types of nonprofit NGOs—client affinity groups, social service clubs, nonprofit firms and broad-based private charities. NGOs of all four types may be indigenous or may be the local affiliate of an international organisation. These tradeoffs can be best understood by considering the two types of organisation at either end of the spectrum. Because the management and staff of a client affinity group is typically drawn from and selected by the client group it is serving, this type of NGO will have the most credibility with its clients.

Furthermore, to the extent that the services for which the government pays the organisation are perceived by its members as in their interest, the clients will themselves monitor its performance, greatly reducing government monitoring costs. For these reasons, client affinity groups can be very cost-effective in delivering highly differentiated services, such as peer counselling of sex workers.

However, the government's ability to delegate to a client affinity group is limited by the fact that the group's interests and objectives will sometimes diverge from those of the general public. For example, it might not be a good idea to subcontract to a client affinity group of sex workers the collection of data on the proportion of its members who are HIV-positive, since the group might perceive that publication of such a number would be against its best interest.

Moreover, some of the members of the affinity group may have socially unacceptable objectives that could be cross-subsidised from government resources. Thus, the divergence of objectives between the client affinity group and the government implies that a service contract with this type of organisation will entail a risk of resource diversion toward the group's own objectives. Addressing this problem will increase monitoring costs. Examples of client affinity groups that attain international recognition and receive international funding are multiplying.

At the other end of the spectrum are the broad-based private charities. These organisations may be religious or secular but typically represent a large body of dues-paying members. Therefore, their constituency mirrors an important portion of the entire public, those who are willing to contribute regularly for charitable causes. Except for divergences due to religious belief, the interests of this mainstream constituency are likely to conform quite closely to those of the general public. However, private charities may not have credibility with all of the subpopulations that the government wishes to reach with its message and thus might be less effective delivering services to them.

Two other types of nonprofit NGOs fall between the affinity group and the large private charity. Social service clubs are local charitable organisations typically composed of middle class and elite community members who volunteer their time in order to improve their community. Their direct constituency, to whom they are primarily accountable, is their peer group within their own community. Social service clubs may be able to establish trust in client groups because service providers live in the same community with the clients and are volunteering their time.

The most sophisticated nonprofit firms are like the profit-oriented in that they can draw on the best national expertise and be held accountable to international standards. But nonprofit firms can, with greater ease and legitimacy than for-profit firms, develop a constituency, independent funding sources and their own agenda of objectives. However, the nonprofit firm typically is constrained by a much smaller constituency, perhaps consisting only of the members of its board of directors and their immediate acquaintances.

How well have governments done in delegating preventive or mitigating service delivery to NGOs? A program in Burkina Faso, one of the four West African nations with a generalised epidemic, offers an example of how government and NGOs acting in concert can extend the reach of their AIDS prevention and mitigation efforts, achieving better quality and access than if either had acted alone. The project, which is supported by the World Bank, seeks to increase the use of condoms and other contraceptives and change, behaviours that facilitate the spread of STDs. The government and NGOs share responsibility and costs.

Government roles include providing supplies at a subsidised rate; launching a national media campaign to promote the purchase of condoms; and teaching traditional healers to fill prescriptions, diagnose STDs and refer cases to health clinics. Treatment of STDs will be handled primarily by NGOs, which are both nonprofit and for-profit firms; NGOs will also provide training to traditional healers. Both NGOs and public clinics will provide free condoms to people with high-risk behaviour.

The government has also provided encouragement and access to grant money for NGOs to enable them to offer additional services. This type of collaboration lays the foundation for increased coordination in the future between the two actors and fosters an environment of trust. The largest and most elaborate effort to subcontract AIDS services to NGOs is probably the annual competition for service grants in Brazil. Supported by a World Bank loan, the program has funded all four types of nonprofit NGOs, including client affinity groups such as an association of transvestites in Rio de Janeiro and nonprofit firms such as a university-affiliated research center in Sao Paulo.

Clients have included children, haemophiliacs, pregnant women, feminists, transvestites, prostitutes, drug users, prisoners, truck drivers and men who have sex with men. While grant competitions are managed centrally by an NGO liaison office attached to the Ministry of Health in Brasilia, state and municipal as well as federal government agencies provide complementary funding to and collaborate actively in the execution of, funded programs. In the recent evaluation of this program, only 7 per cent of the 111 current grantee NGOs were deemed to be falling short of their project objectives and only 2 per cent were having serious difficulties reaching their target populations.

The financial control mechanisms employed by the liaison office, which include an annual visit to each grantee and audit of its accounts, has identified serious mismanagement in connection with less than 1 per cent of projects.

The availability of a set of standard, transparent, internationally recognised procedures for governments to follow in delegating service provision to NGOs could greatly facilitate government-NGO cooperation and minimize the disappointment of all parties concerned. AIDS donors, NGOs, government policymakers and indeed the entire international health community would benefit from studies of the costs and effectiveness of alternative procedures for identifying effective NGOs to be service providers and for monitoring their performance.

Donor support for national AIDS programs is important and, in a nascent epidemic, often critical; yet there are other crucial activities in which donors have a greater comparative advantage and a clearer public economics mandate. Because the benefits of prevention programs accrue primarily to a country's own population, all but the poorest national governments can and should finance a significant share of these costs. In contrast, donors are in a unique position to mobilise international support for the creation and dissemination of knowledge and technology that is transferable across countries.

Although AIDS was first diagnosed in 1981, a systematic international and national response to the epidemic was not evident until the late 1980s. In many parts of the world, NGOs led the way in providing care and prevention services for individuals and communities affected by the epidemic. The incremental and relatively limited response of WHO in the early years has been attributed to resistance by many member states to addressing the problem of HIV/AIDS. The establishment of the WHO Global Programme on AIDS (GPA) in 1987 helped to generate momentum for global prevention and mitigation efforts; that same year the UN General Assembly adopted a resolution encouraging UN agencies and other members of the UN family to initiate their own HIV/AIDS activities.

During its early years GPA focused on helping national governments develop strategies to curb the spread of the epidemic. The year GPA was established, 170 countries requested assistance; by 1989 GPA had helped 151 countries to establish national AIDS programs, 102 countries to develop short term (6 to 12 month) plans and 30 countries to develop medium-term (3 to 5 year) plans. Largely as the result of the prodigious efforts of GPA, almost all countries today have national AIDS programs; most of them were formed between 1985 and 1990. Meanwhile, in response to the UN General Assembly Resolution, UNDP, UNICEF, UNFPA and UNESCO developed a joint HIV/AIDS strategy document that specified the resources and staffing that each would allocate to combating the epidemic. UNDP played the most prominent role, devoting 2.1 per cent of overall agency resources and 0.43 per cent of overall agency staff.

Other multilaterals also initiated AIDS programs. In 1987 the European Union established the AIDS Task Force in order to fund AIDs-related programs in developing countries. The World Bank, which made its first loan exclusively to combat AIDS in 1986, had financed 61 projects in 41 countries, for a total commitment of $632 million by the end of 1996 making it the largest source of funds for confronting HIV/AIDS.

In the late 1980s, the wealthier donor countries, in addition to making contributions to the GPA and providing support through the other multilaterals, also launched their own bilateral HIV/AIDS programs. By 1993 the largest of these was the US program; launched in 1988, it includes the centrally funded AIDS Control and Prevention Project (AIDSCAP) as well as other activities initiated and funded by country USAID missions. Other countries with large bilateral AIDS programs include Canada and Norway;

Denmark, Germany, the Netherlands, Sweden, the United kingdom, Japan, Belgium, France, Australia and Switzerland.

Under the leadership of the GPA, many national plans were written, many AIDS interventions were launched and many national leaders became aware of the severity of the AIDS epidemic. For the first time, senior policymakers discussed high-risk sexual behaviour and how governments should respond. However, the epidemic continued to spread. In the early 1990s a group of member states, especially the donor governments then funding the GPA, became concerned that, as a part of WHO, it had insufficient mandate to coordinate the expanding efforts against the epidemic across the UN system.

The donor community perceived that the GPA was unable to restrain donors from competing vigorously with one another instead of cooperating around a mutually agreed plan of action and came to believe it necessary to create a specialised international institution with an explicit mandate to coordinate the work of the other UN agencies at the country level. As a result they worked with UNDP, the World Bank and other multilaterals to create a new special-purpose UN program dedicated uniquely to combating AIDS.

The Joint UN Programme on AIDS, widely known as UNAIDS, officially began operations on January 1, 1996. It is based in Geneva and works most closely with its six cosponsoring agencies: WHO, UNDP, UNICEF, UNFPA, UNESCO and the World Bank. It is governed by a Programme Coordinating Board (PCB) of 22 member states and 6 cosponsors, plus, for the first time in the UN system, 5 rotating nonvoting representatives of NGOs.

The PCB has assigned UNAIDS four roles: first, policy development and research, which are to account for a larger share of UNAIDS activities than it did of the GPA's; second, like the GPA before it, UNAIDS is to take the lead among UN agencies in providing technical support to national AIDS programs around the world; third, the program is committed more formally to advocacy on behalf of HIV/AIDS prevention and mitigation than was the GPA; and finally,

UNAIDS is charged with the difficult task of coordination of its cosponsors and of other UN agencies.

In this last role, it can potentially address the needs described in the next section by serving as a forum within which multilateral and bilateral donors can agree to donate more to AIDS research, prevention and control than they otherwise would. Since cooperation with other donors at the country level entails substantially increased costs to each donor and deprives each of being able to claim sole credit for supporting the government on a specific activity, the incentives for such cooperation are weak. Since UNAIDS lacks the power to enforce cooperation from its co-sponsoring multilaterals, much less from the bilaterals, the hope for this form of donor cooperation lies in the good will of the staff of the various donors working at the country level—perhaps reinforced by the insistence of the national government.

The current and future magnitude of HIV's contribution to the infectious disease burden within industrial countries' borders provides them with two reasons to spend money on HIV control in the low income countries. First, any lessons learned about how to slow the spread of the epidemic, whether through behavioural modification or technological advances, are potentially applicable at home. Second, because HIV is infectious and the higher-income countries exchange thousands of tourists and attract thousands of legal and illegal immigrants to their shores every year, a reduction in HIV prevalence in low-income countries has a secondary effect of protecting the citizens of higher-income countries. Evidence suggests that countries are already aware of these arguments: the five countries that provide the most support to the global effort against AIDS also receive the most immigrants.

A free-rider problem, however, threatens to prevent the donor countries from voluntarily donating as much to the AIDS effort in developing countries as the abolition of the epidemic would in fact be worth to them. Because it suffers from this international free-rider problem, the effort to combat AIDS can be viewed as an international public good.

Another good on which it is easy to free-ride is new technical information, such as that generated by frontier medical research on treatment of AIDS and opportunistic illnesses, AIDS vaccines, or, to the degree that the results are transferable across countries, by operations research on the best way to market condoms to the people most likely to contract and spread HIV. The solution to problems of local or national public goods is typically government intervention.

At the international level, the United Nations is a forum for such negotiation and persuasion. Through it, countries can potentially be persuaded to donate their "fair share" to international public goods, such as AIDS control. Thus from the public economics point of view, it is not surprising that donor countries have been willing to donate to AIDS control and to research on AIDS. However, given the free-rider problem, it is unlikely that the donor countries have committed as much as it would be in their joint best interest to provide.

Information that can be generalised beyond the country in which it is produced can originate in either the social or the physical sciences. The medical and social sciences of epidemiology, sociology, economics and operations research are necessary to track the epidemic and to learn what sort of interventions prevent the most secondary cases of HIV infection per government dollar spent. Applied social science research offers the greatest hope for immediately slowing the spread of AIDS and of improving the well-being of the hardest-hit survivors. The biological sciences, including microbiology, immunology and virology, are making slow progress toward a vaccine and a cure. However, market imperfections mean that only a small share of biomedical research is designed to produce products or knowledge that will benefit low-income countries.

WHO's ad hoc Committee on Health Research estimates that 95 per cent of spending on health research and development is directed toward solving health problems that mostly affect the richest 10 per cent of the worlds population; only 5 per cent of such spending is directed toward the diseases that account for most of the disease burden of the remaining 90 per cent of the world's population. An important role of governments, especially of donors, is to tilt incentives for medical research somewhat more in favour of the low-income countries.

A third important type of public good is the international institution that enables a group of countries to coordinate their efforts in their mutual best interests. Two types of international institutions are relevant to the AIDS epidemic: those among low-income countries in a region and those that bring poor and high-income countries together in a common struggle against HIV/AIDS. Information from the social sciences on behavioural interventions. Any successful preventive intervention among individuals who are very likely to spread the virus will produce positive spillover effects for the host country, in the form of reduced secondary transmission, which to some degree will also benefit other countries. But the most valuable output of such an intervention for the outside world is knowledge that can be applied in other countries.

Donors who fund behavioural interventions have a responsibility to ensure that the opportunities for the generation of new knowledge that arise from such programs are not wasted. Although the imperative to learn from interventions seems self-evident, surprisingly little is being done in this regard. Recent literature reviews found that publicly available written evaluations exist for only about 10 per cent of donor-funded interventions. Worse, of the few hundred published studies, very few were conducted with sufficient thoroughness to determine whether or not the intervention actually changed the risk behaviour or HIV incidence.

The reviewers noted many deficiencies in the available studies. In some cases the lack of baseline data made it impossible to know whether a measured difference between a control and experimental group was due to differences in the two groups present before the intervention. In others, baseline data were collected but there was no control group against which the intervention group could be compared.

Few studies attempted to determine whether changes in behaviour were due to the intervention or to a placebo effect arising from existence of the study. Differences between the standards of knowledge for pharmaceutical products and those for behavioural interventions against HIV are striking. Since pharmaceutical products can be patented, private firms have a strong incentive to win the race to the market with a new drug. Governments have responded by requiring that companies prove the safety and the efficacy of new drugs, typically at a cost of millions of dollars. These sums are spent even on such relatively minor drugs as a new headache pill in order to ensure very high standards. The government does not hesitate to require such expenditures, knowing that firms will spend this money on any drug they think will pass the market test.

In contrast, preventive interventions that have the potential of producing far more public benefits, in the form of secondary HIV infections averted, are held to much weaker standards. Since these kinds of interventions can not be patented and they produce positive externalities, the public sector typically must finance them. If governments held themselves to standards as rigorous as those they set for pharmaceutical manufacturers, HIV prevention interventions would be forced to meet standards of rigorous design and data collection methods that would enable the public to learn whether an intervention will be safe and efficacious in subsequent application.

Some observers, aware of these prohibitive costs and pessimistic about the prospects for successful behavioural interventions, believe that the only hope for reducing the impact of HIV on low-income countries is a vaccine. But vaccine research of all types faces serious impediments. These include the increasing complexity and expense of vaccine research, the need to sell perhaps 40 million doses before production processes attain economies of scale; the inability of people in developing countries to afford expensive vaccines; and, perhaps most serious, companies' vulnerability to damage claims in the millions of dollars, if even one dose of a vaccine causes the disease it was designed to prevent.

Partly as a result of these impediments, worldwide public and private sector investment in vaccine development totalled a mere $160 million in 1993 compared with an estimated $1.3 billion spent on other approaches to prevent HIV infection and about $5 billion spent on HIV-related health care. In order to achieve the substantial international public benefits of vaccines for the diseases of the developing world, governments must play a role. The May 1997 announcement of a US goal to produce an effective AIDS vaccine within ten years as a US national goal is welcome news not only for people in the US but for people everywhere, including developing countries.

International institutions can produce international public goods. We noted above that the United Nations and other multilateral organisations can provide forums in which countries can persuade one another to contribute more than they otherwise would to the production of an international public good. Two additional types of international institutions that could solve specific kinds of international free-rider problems are private-public alliances for health research and regional cooperation bodies.

Public-private alliance for health research

WHO's Ad Hoc Committee on Health Research has recently proposed a "Health Product Development Alliance" between the public and private sectors whose mandate would be tightly focused on the development of a limited number of products for major causes of disease burden that are currently neglected by existing efforts. Such an alliance would use a variety of approaches to improve the incentives for private firms to develop pharmaceutical and other health care products urgently needed in developing countries. These mechanisms, some of which require changes in the tax codes and legislation of participating countries, include:

- direct support for the costs of the early stages of product development.
- analysis of the potential market for a specific new product that would primarily benefit people in the lowest-income countries.

— tax relief and or streamlined regulatory controls for the development of products for low-income countries.
— worldwide tax breaks for pharmaceutical companies and extended periods during which they have the exclusive right to sell the drug.
— advance guarantee of a market for a health product that meets certain objectively verifiable criteria.

The last idea is a particularly innovative approach to solving the incentive problem. One way to implement the idea would be for one or more low-income countries with a specific disease problem not being adequately tackled by biomedical research to offer to buy a large quantity of the first drug or other medical product that meets precise specifications, regardless of the identity of the developer.

To be credible, this offer would be guaranteed by a consortium of international donors and lenders. The total financial package could include, for example, grants from bilateral donors and a mixture of soft or market-rate loans from multilateral institutions or even commercial lenders. In the purest form of the guarantee, none of this financing would be released until the desired product was approved by independent testing laboratories. Only then, as the culmination of a period of research and development that might last as long as five or ten years, would the financial instruments be executed, the donor contributions delivered, the international loans disbursed and the delivery and distribution of the product initiated.

The most urgently needed anti-AIDS technology—a vaccine to protect against HIV infection—is already the subject of a public-private partnership. Established in 1996, the International AIDS Vaccine Initiative (IAVI) is the first attempt to organise a health product development alliance along the lines recommended by the Ad Hoc Committee on Health Research. First proposed by the Rockefeller Foundation, the IAVI has attracted support from the Merieux Foundation, UNAIDS and the World Bank.

Its mandate is to accelerate the development of HIV vaccines appropriate for worldwide use by reducing obstacles to vaccine development and filling gaps in the current effort. In 1997, IAVI's first full year of operation, participants expected to devote a total of $2 million to $4 million in direct support of research on an AIDS vaccine. In light of the US initiative to produce an AIDS vaccine, the challenge to IAVI will be to assure that vaccine development programs do not neglect the needs of low-income countries, where 90 per cent of HIV infections occur.

Other important potential applications for a public-private alliance in the AIDS arena lie in the development of vaginal microbicides and virucides, which would allow a woman to protect herself from HIV infection without asking her partner to wear a condom. Poor women in developing countries are often at a particular disadvantage in negotiating condom use with their partners; yet these same women are also most likely to lack the purchasing power to buy a vaginal virucide.

By guaranteeing the market, a public-private alliance would provide an incentive for pharmaceutical companies to develop such products. Public-private partnerships could also offer incentives for development of reliable, inexpensive diagnostic tests for STDs such as chlamydia, which are prevalent in developing countries and accelerate the spread of HIV and to stimulate research that would lower the cost of antiretroviral therapies.

Interest group and AIDS policy

Many groups with divergent interests affect the design and implementation of HIV/AIDS policy and the mix of groups and their relative strength changes over the course of the epidemic. At the outset, few groups are concerned. However, as the epidemic progresses, the number of interest groups increases and the politics of AIDS becomes ever more complex. Early in the epidemic, physicians and medical suppliers have an interest in learning how to treat AIDS and how to protect the safety of health care workers from needle sticks and other accidental infection on the job.

A group that emerges at about the same time is people infected with HIV. Although the number of these individuals is initially small and they may at the outset lack political influence, they are often highly motivated to lobby government, since their very lives may depend on persuading the government to subsidise AIDS treatment and care. As the epidemic spreads, the size of this group and its potential to influence government policy increase. Often overlapping with this group are individuals who practice high-risk behaviour but who are not infected—or hope they are not infected. Although these people have a strong interest in government-subsidised prevention for themselves, in the early stages of the epidemic they are rarely well organised enough to lobby on their own behalf.

Yet increasingly the AIDS epidemic has induced people with the highest risk behaviour to organise in order to promote their interests. Furthermore, NGOs working on HIV prevention and AIDS care become advocates for the populations they serve. Finally, as the number of AIDS cases increases, insurance providers and employers will become concerned about rising health care costs and increased sickness and death among employees.

At all stages of the epidemic, the largest interest group is the one least motivated to learn about the issues or lobby on its own behalf: the general public of HIV-negative individuals who rarely practice risky behaviour. Like most of those with riskier behaviour, these people at low risk have an interest in marriage, in conceiving and raising healthy children and in seeing them married, all without the risk of HIV infection. Although not themselves suffering from AIDS, in a generalised epidemic these people find that the price of health care has greatly increased because of higher demand and increased costs. Some of these people are the poor who have never suffered an HIV infection or death but nevertheless need help in order to escape poverty. Some suffer dangerous chronic diseases other than HIV, such as cancer, kidney disease or diabetes and cannot afford the treatment to keep themselves alive.

To be truly democratic, a society must find ways—for example, opinion polls or elections—for the many with a small interest in an issue to express their views inexpensively and influence the course of events. Politicians facing a ballot box have an incentive to seek the opinions of ordinary people and consider these together with the views of smaller, more vocal interest groups. A government that is responsive to the nation's political leadership will follow suit.

In the case of HIV/AIDS, the policies that will best protect the average citizen are not necessarily popular. Politicians and government officials, who may themselves be unsure of the best policies for confronting the epidemic, have the difficult task of explaining to the public why taxes should be spent subsidising condoms and STD treatment for prostitutes and clean needles for injecting drug users. Conservative social and religious groups, perhaps not fully appreciating the great harm that can arise from failing to prevent the spread of HIV, may oppose efforts to reduce the risks involved in commercial sex or injecting drug use, or to encourage condom use generally, out of concern that these efforts will encourage behaviour they regard as immoral.

An authoritative case study of Thailand highlights other political problems that can arise in designing and implementing an effective response. In the second half of the 1980s, as evidence that HIV was spreading rapidly among Thai sex workers and injecting drug users accumulated, a government official insisted that the situation was under control: "The general public need not be alarmed. Thai-to-Thai transmission is not in evidence." In keeping with this sanguine view, the government spent only $180,000 on HIV prevention in 1988 (the GPA committed $500,000 to Thailand that same year). The study suggests that during this period of democratic rule, in a pattern reminiscent of that described by Ibsen in Norway 100 years before, "high-level cabinet pressure was brought to bear on the ministry of public health not to publicise the emergence of increasing HIV in the population".

Although Thai national funding increased to $2.6 million by 1990 (and donor funding reached $3.4 million), the government did not initiate a high-profile, aggressive campaign to control HIV until 1991-92, when the country was led by Premier Anand Panyarachun, who had been appointed by the leaders of a military coup. The new prime minister took several important steps that have since been credited with helping to slow and perhaps reverse the epidemic in Thailand. First, he shifted control of the AIDS control program out of the Ministry of Public Health to the Office of the Prime Minister, giving it added political clout. Second, he increased the budget almost 20-fold, to $44 million in 1993. Perhaps most important, he initiated the "100 per cent condom program" focused on brothels.

Since then Thai funding to AIDS control has continued to increase, reaching more than $80 million in 1996, a sum equivalent to more than one-quarter of the entire international donor commitment to AIDS control in developing countries that year. The high-profile campaign was initially unpopular with the influential tourism industry and tourism indeed temporarily declined. However, once AIDS had a prominent place on the national agenda, opposition to the measures gradually faded-out and support increased. "There were too many vested interests in maintaining the high status of the national AIDS program to make a policy reversal," the case study noted. "In particular, the enormous budget allocated to the HIV/AIDS prevention and control campaign was vigorously coveted by a wide-range of participants".

Thus, the policy situation in Thailand had come full circle, from one in which special interest groups used their influence to oppose a vigorous prevention policy, to one in which the participants in the prevention program assumed the role of vested interests in sustaining it. Since all programs that involve significant public expenditure develop their own constituencies, policymakers must be careful at the outset to initiate programs that are in the interest of the general public, as appears to have been the case in Mexico and Thailand.

Donor assistance and public consensus

Although the politics of AIDS will differ greatly across countries, bilateral donors and multilateral organisations can help to encourage public consensus on effective, low-cost responses to HIV through direct funding and through a judicious use of encouragement and conditionality. For countries that are still in the nascent stage, where citizens are not sufficiently aware of the epidemic to support funding activities from public revenue, donor funding can be critical in gathering surveillance data or establishing a demonstration project.

Sometimes donors can require certain actions as a condition of the receipt of an aid package. However, the leverage afforded by conditionality is often quite limited and may depend on all donors agreeing to the desirability of a given condition. Conditionality is more likely to work if the government intends to carry out the action in any case but has not yet made it high enough priority to get it accomplished. One example of the effective application of conditionality occurred during negotiations of the $70 million World Bank loan to India. In 1991 the government's initial posture was that there was no need for specific interventions with sex workers and their clients in Indian cities. One influential government figure asserted that "in India AIDS is not sexually transmitted."

As a result of a position taken jointly by GPA and the World Bank, the government of India agreed to double the size of its proposed AIDS program to include interventions with those most likely to contract and spread HIV, to be implemented by NGOs. Since then the extent of the sexually transmitted AIDS epidemic in India has become obvious to the highest levels of government, as evidenced in a 1997 speech by Prime Minister Deva Gowda. Attention has turned from whether interventions with those who practice the riskiest behaviour are necessary to how best to implement them. These instances suggest that donors can significantly improve the timing and quality of country-level responses to HIV/AIDS.

Donors have often waited until AIDS has moved beyond the nascent stage before providing support. Although the data suggest that multilateral institutions are more likely than bilateral donors to direct resources to countries at the concentrated stage of the epidemic, neither supports countries sufficiently at the nascent stage, when the largest benefits can be achieved with the smallest expenditure.

As the understanding of the epidemic increases, a growing number of individuals in developing countries are demonstrating such leadership. To mention just three examples: the speech by Indian Prime Minister Deve Gowda naming HIV/AIDS as a national health problem helped to overcome the idea that India was somehow not threatened by the virus. Zambian President Kenneth Kaunda, in acknowledging publicly that his son had died of AIDS, helped to energize his country's response to the ravages of a widespread epidemic. Finally, Marina Mahathir, daughter of Malaysian Prime Minister Mahathir Mohamad and the president of the Malaysian AIDS Council, a non-governmental organisation, has spoken out in her own country and internationally for greater political commitment to mobilising the resources necessary for effective prevention. Some of the most compelling advocates of an effective response to the epidemic are people who are themselves infected with HIV.

With assistance from UNICEF, the Initiative sponsors lectures in schools and communities across Uganda highlighting personal testimonials of hundreds of people infected with HIV. A 90-minute television documentary on Lutaaya's struggle with AIDS released in 1990 reached millions of television viewers around the world. But a person need not be a celebrity prior to infection for personal testimony to have a powerful impact. Perhaps the most courageous individuals are otherwise ordinary people who, after becoming infected, step forward to acknowledge their disease and, in the face of discrimination and persecution and with very limited personal financial resources to draw upon, speak out for a more effective public response. All these individuals serve as a powerful example to those who meet them, a few become nationally known.

Each types of organisations has particular strengths and that for an effective global response to HIV/AIDS, all of these groups, plus countless exemplary individuals, must work toward a common goal of overcoming the epidemic. Governments have the unique responsibility for coordinating their country's overall response to the epidemic. As part of that responsibility, many governments, especially in developing countries, should take on greater responsibility for basic epidemiological surveillance and prevention activities. NGOs have often played an important role in prodding governments into action; governments that select appropriate NGO partners can often greatly increase their reach, especially in working with marginalised groups to help people who practice the riskiest behaviour to protect themselves and others. Donors and the multilateral institutions they support have provided significant financing and other assistance for all of these efforts. But donors need to do a better job of focusing attention and resources on countries where the epidemic has yet to attract policymakers' attention, especially countries with nascent epidemics, where prevention is most cost-effective.

Moreover, international donors have the unique ability to mobilise financing and other support for international public goods, such as evaluation of alternative approaches to preventing HIV and mitigating the impact of AIDS, as well as research on a vaccine that would work in developing countries. Such efforts are in the donors' own best interest, as well as the interest of developing countries and deserve much greater attention and support. Finally, donors have the responsibility to coordinate their activities at the country level, both among themselves and with the national government.

Although there are no easy solutions to the technical and political problems posed by the HIV/AIDS epidemic, examples from countries around the world offer hope that people of good will, working together, can overcome this global epidemic.

Over the past two decades the human immunodeficiency virus has spread silently throughout the world, profoundly affecting the lives of men and women, their families and societies. It has not respected international boundaries or spared the elite. By the time that researchers understood how HIV spreads, how it can be prevented and the behaviours that put people at risk, HIV had already infected millions of adults in the industrial and developing world. In the hardest-hit countries in Sub-Saharan Africa, poverty, illiteracy, poor health, low status of women and political instability fuelled its spread. By the time East African health authorities identified the mysterious "slim" disease as AIDS in the early 1980s, HIV had already widely infected those with the riskiest behaviour and had a firm foothold in the general population.

On the medical frontier there have been many advances, but there is still no vaccine for HIV and no cure for AIDS. Medical researchers have succeeded in substantially prolonging the lives of some people living with HIV and AIDS in industrial countries. However, these treatments are still very expensive, they are not always successful and no one knows for how long they prolong life. The costs of these new therapies are so high and the requirements for their implementation are so demanding that they are simply not feasible in low-income countries and would bankrupt the health systems of middle-income countries.

HIV is not spread easily and that it can be prevented through behavioural change. Other STDs signal risky behaviour and preventing or treating these STDs can slow HIV transmission rates. Low-cost-effective interventions to prevent HIV/AIDS in poor countries now known to exist. Behaviour change has reduced incidence of HIV among specific groups in countries as diverse as Australia and Thailand. And there are many opportunities to alleviate suffering and prolong the lives of HIV-infected people in developing countries, for example, through low-cost treatments of common opportunities infections, particularly tuberculosis. We can also learn from the policy mistakes of the past. No country, rich or poor, is insulated from the risk of HIV.

Behavioural change must focus first on people with high-risk behaviour who are most likely to become infected and unknowingly infect others. But discrimination against such individuals makes behavioural change more difficult and inhibits efforts to cope with the impact of AIDS. Experience has also shown that active government involvement is crucial if AIDS is to be overcome. Only governments have the means and mandate to finance the public goods necessary for the monitoring and control of the disease—epidemiological surveillance, basic research on sexual behaviour, information collection for identifying high-risk groups and evaluation of the costs and effectiveness of interventions.

Private individuals left to their own devices would not invest adequately in these activities. Governments also have a unique responsibility to intervene to reduce the negative externalities of high-risk behaviour, while preventing discrimination that would inhibit behavioural change. Without these government efforts, those at high risk of contracting and spreading HIV are unlikely to reduce risky behaviours enough from the perspective of the rest of society. The government role extends to ensuring equity in access to HIV prevention and treatment for the most destitute.

Other key functions that most governments are already attempting to perform can also make an important contribution to slowing the spread of HIV: promoting labour-intensive economic growth to reduce poverty, assuring basic social services, law and order, human and property rights; and protecting the poor. Investing in female schooling and ensuring equal rights for women in employment, inheritance, divorce and child custody proceedings are part of this broader mandate.

These policies yield large development benefits in their own right but are also important for preventing an HIV epidemic and coping with its impact. Reform of health systems, as outlined in the World Development Report 1993, will improve the efficiency of health care delivery, including HIV and STD prevention and will reduce the impact of AIDS on the health system. In areas where there is a severe epidemic and targeted poverty reduction programs already exist, these can often be combined with efforts to ease the impact on surviving household members, especially children, in the most destitute families that suffer a prime-age adult death.

Certain policies can work, yet developing countries face many financial, political and managerial obstacles to implementing them. Financial resources are scarce. In low-income countries, annual health spending from public and private sources averages only $16 per person. This is one-tenth the resources available in middle-income countries and only 0.7 per cent of the $2,300 per capita annual health spending in high-income countries. Many developing country governments also have limited capability to implement complex or multifaceted programs. The World Development Report 1997 makes a compelling case that the government role must be matched with its capability.

In fighting the spread of HIV and mitigating the impact of AIDS, developing country governments will be most effective if they focus their financial and other resources on a limited set of feasible activities that have the potential to be highly cost-effective. Governments can sometimes expand their effectiveness by involving the private sector, reputable NGOs, those most severely affected and decentralised community organisations in the design and implementation of high-priority HIV/AIDS prevention activities. However, coordination and management of these activities can also stretch the capabilities of government.

OPPORTUNITIES TO CHANGE THE COURSE OF EPIDEMIC

Epidemiological models predict that between 1996 and 2001, between 10 and 30 million new infections will occur in developing countries. But the future of the epidemic is not carved in stone. One reason that such projections are very uncertain is that nobody knows the extent to which individuals, especially those most likely to contract and spread HIV, will change their behaviour in response to the virus. Concerted, focused action in developing countries, where more than 90 per cent of HIV infections occur, can save millions of lives.

Preventing nascent epidemics

Public action can make the greatest difference for the 2.4 billion people who live in areas where the epidemic is nascent. Developing areas with nascent epidemics include half of the world population, two-thirds of the population of developing countries and nearly 40 per cent of the population of low-income countries. Half of India, all of

China except Yunnan Province, Indonesia, the Philippines, most of Eastern Europe, the former Soviet Union, North Africa, a third of the countries in Latin America and the Caribbean are at this stage. In these areas, HIV has not yet spread widely even among those whose behaviour puts them at risk. But countries with nascent epidemics cannot assume that they will never be affected; every country that now has a generalised AIDS epidemic went through a phase of denial that gave the virus time to gain a foothold. These nascent-stage areas present an enormous opportunity for governments and donors to prevent an HIV epidemic by intervening actively and early.

Epidemiological surveillance of those who practice the riskiest behaviour and studies of risky behaviours in the general population and specific subgroups have high payoff at this stage. An HIV/AIDS epidemic can be pre-empted, for little cost, by promotion of safe injecting behaviour among injecting drug users and of safe sex and STD prevention through condom use among those with high levels of sexual activity.

Prevention efforts focused on those who practice the riskiest behaviour may be politically controversial, especially if such efforts are perceived by some constituencies as facilitating antisocial or immoral behaviour. Policymakers who encounter such opposition have an obligation to make clear that preventing infections among those with risky behaviour is the best way to protect everyone.

Developing countries with concentrated epidemics—where HIV prevalence exceeds 5 per cent in one or more groups with high-risk behaviour but not in the general population—are a diverse group of low and middle-income countries, with a variety of risk factors. In Latin America, Ukraine, Yunnan province of China, much of Indochina and the northeast of India, the epidemic has reached concentrated levels among injecting drug users; in many countries in Latin America, the epidemic has also reached concentrated levels among homosexual and bisexual men. Once HIV has reached high levels among those who are most likely to contract and spread the virus, containing the epidemic is difficult and requires drastic action—but is nonetheless possible. Thailand undertook such a massive effort when injecting drug users and prostitutes were discovered to have high infection rates. A policy of heavily subsidised condom promotion and STD treatment programs for prostitutes and others with high-risk behaviour, supplemented by widespread dissemination of information to the general population, brought down the prevalence of HIV among military conscripts within a few years.

Not all countries have the same institutional setup or implementing capacity as Thailand. Each country will have to find its own way. But whatever tactics are adopted, the underlying strategy of massive interventions to change the behaviour of those most likely to contract and spread HIV is crucial.

Adapting this strategy successfully will require better information about the cost-effectiveness of alternative interventions to prevent the spread of HIV. Research documenting the effectiveness of such interventions in preventing secondary infections can be very valuable in generating and sustaining support for these measures. Governments also have a role in ensuring that basic information about HIV is presented to the general public in ways that will minimise irrational fear and persecution of individuals who are infected with HIV or thought to engage in high-risk behaviour, since such responses make it harder to reach those with risky behaviour and encourage safer behaviour.

As people infected early in the epidemic begin to get sick and die from AIDS, governments will face growing pressure to spend public resources on care and treatment. Responding to these needs compassionately, while keeping them in perspective with the many other pressing human needs and demands upon public resources, is one of the most difficult challenges posed by the epidemic. Pressure for spending for AIDS care and treatment will be stronger in a generalised epidemic, when the disease has spread into the general population and people infected with HIV are a large and highly motivated constituency. By then, subsidies begun during the concentrated stage may be unsustainable and yet very difficult to withdraw politically. The concentrated stage of the epidemic is therefore the time when policymakers and their constituents need to consider how government can best respond to the medical needs of people with HIV.

The fair response in terms is to offer the same level of subsidy for the care and treatment of people with AIDS as for the care and treatment of people with other diseases that are expensive and difficult to treat. Denying care to individuals simply because they have HIV/AIDS is unjust to those who are infected and to their families. By the same token, providing a higher level of subsidy for AIDS care than for other illnesses is also unfair to the majority of people who are not infected with HIV. Choices about the appropriate overall level of public subsidies for health care will vary across societies.

Governments and their constituents should be aware, however, that high subsidy levels will be extremely difficult to sustain in the face of a large epidemic. Since it is unfair and impractical to deny care and treatment subsidies to people with HIV while providing them to people with other illnesses, any changes in subsidy levels should apply equally to the HIV infected and the uninfected. Policymakers need also be aware that the care and treatment of AIDS, in sharp contrast to preventive interventions focused on those most likely to spread HIV, is primarily a private rather than a public good: most of the benefits of the care and treatment of AIDS accrue to the person who receives the care.

There are important exceptions to this general rule. Treating tuberculosis, STDs and other infectious diseases in people with HIV can prevent these infections from spreading to others, including people who are HIV-negative; these "externalities" are a sound rationale for public funding of such treatments, regardless of whether the recipient of the treatment has HIV.

Similarly, outreach programs that include care for those infected with HIV who practice high-risk behaviour may be a justifiable use of public funds if the program results in behaviour changes that reduce the spread of the virus.

Often, however, demands for publicly funded care and treatment threaten to drain scarce resources that could have been used for preventing new infections.

Countries with a generalised epidemic will face two related sets of challenges: establishing or maintaining prevention programs focused on those most likely to contract and spread HIV, while expanding prevention efforts to those with somewhat lower risk of transmitting the virus; and mitigating the impact of AIDS sickness and death, especially among the poor. Except for Botswana and South Africa, all countries that currently have generalised epidemics are low-income, with 1995 per capita income of $765 or less. Scarce financial and managerial resources mean that these governments must be especially vigilant in implementing the most cost-effective prevention programs.

Although prevention measure for the general population become increasingly cost-effective as prevalence rises, interventions for those practising the riskiest behaviour continue to have the greatest impact on incidence per dollar spent and must be maintained even as prevention programs are expanded to others condom social marketing programs and other forms of prevention subsidies aimed at poor people who would otherwise be unable to afford to protect themselves are an appropriate government response at this stage, where resources are available. But these programs are no substitute for reaching the highest-risk groups. Indeed, one of the greatest threats to effective prevention in generalised epidemics is pressure to divert resources from highly targeted cost-effective interventions to politically popular interventions with lower cost-effectiveness.

Even where prevention measures are very effective, declines in prevalence will occur only gradually, as people already infected die and are succeeded by younger cohorts. But declines in incidence—the number of new infections—can be achieved relatively quickly, even in the face of a generalised epidemic. Recent declines in HIV incidence among young people in Uganda are an encouraging sign that even the worst-hit countries can make progress against the epidemic.

The second challenge to governments in a generalised epidemic is mitigating its impact, especially on the poor. A widespread epidemic will greatly increase the number of households that suffer a prime-age adult death. In poor households, such deaths can have a severe and lasting impact on surviving children, who may suffer further declines in already inadequate nutrition and schooling. But not all households that suffer a prime-age adult death are poor. Indeed, in many of the countries hardest hit by AIDS, while most of those infected may be poor, it is still the case that nonpoor people are more likely to be infected than the poor.

Confronted with demands to finance programs to help households affected by AIDS, policymakers need to balance the needs of poor households hit by AIDS with the needs of other poor households that are more numerous and often poorer. In approaching this task, they should ask two questions: Which households need help most? How best can they be helped? If many households are very poor and children are malnourished and not in school, government's priorities must include such basic development policies as fostering labour-intensive economic growth, improving nutrition levels and increasing school enrolment, especially of girls. Where targeted poverty reduction programs are already in place, modifying these programs to make assistance available to very poor families that suffer a prime-age adult death can help to improve the targeting of assistance to the households that need help most.

CHALLENGES FOR THE INTERNATIONAL COMMUNITY

International donors have been generous in their support for AIDS prevention in developing countries, but their support has not always gone to those interventions that are most cost-effective from the perspective of government. To have the largest impact now on the pandemic, donors need to consider two main strategies.

First, in terms of bilateral and multilateral assistance, donors should support major interventions in countries at the nascent stage of the epidemic, including epidemiological surveillance, surveys of risky behaviour and programs to change behaviour among those who practice the riskiest behaviour. Among countries at the concentrated and generalised stages, particularly the low-income countries, ensuring prevention of infection among those who practice the riskiest behaviour would be the most cost-effective strategy.

Moreover, donor funds could help promote such programs when they might be politically unworkable if openly sponsored by government. With respect to mitigating the tragic impact of AIDS on society, donors must not lose sight of the myriad development problems faced by the low-income countries with generalised epidemics. The AIDS epidemic will increase poverty and will undermine household investments in human capital. Countries with generalised epidemics are therefore likely to need renewed support for core public programs to raise levels of human capital and reduce poverty.

In addition, there may be some scope in specific hard-hit areas for assistance in integrating targeted poverty reduction efforts and AIDS mitigation. However, governments and donors need to be careful that such assistance does not displace household and community efforts to cope or, worse, drain time, energy and money from prevention measures focused on people who practice high-risk behaviour.

The second important strategy for international donors is to finance key international public goods that poor countries cannot afford to support collectively. Two important public goods stand out: knowledge about the costs and impact of interventions on the incidence of HIV in differing environments; and development of vaccines and low-cost preventive medical technologies that will be effective under conditions prevailing in developing countries.

Country after country responded to evidence of the first infections by saying "We are different. AIDS cannot strike us." Each has been proven wrong. When countries discovered that they indeed did have a fatal, sexually transmitted disease spreading rapidly in their midst, one after another responded by cleaning up the blood supply or conducting general awareness campaigns while avoiding or devoting insufficient resources to efforts to encourage safer behaviour among people most likely to contract and spread the virus

But recent history also offers valuable examples of success. Experience demonstrates that enabling people who practice the riskiest behaviour to protect themselves and others can be extraordinarily effective. National policymakers now face the challenge of applying this strategy in the cultural and political context of their own countries.

SELECTED READINGS

Aina, T.A., 1991. Patterns of Bisexuality in Sub-Saharan Africa. In: *Bisexuality and HIV/AIDS: A Global Perspective,* edited by R. Tielman, M. Carballo, and A. Hendriks, Bufallo, NY: Prometheus Books.

American Psychiatric Association (1994). *Diagnostic and Statistical Manual of Mental Disorders* (4th Ed.) (DSM-IV). Washington, DC: Author.

Boyd-Franklin, N., Aleman, J. del C., Jean-Gilles, M. M., & Lewis, S. Y. (1995). Cultural sensitivity and competence. In N. Boyd-Franklin, G. L. Steiner & M. G. Boland (Eds.), *Children, families and HIV/AIDS.* New York: Guilford Press.

Carmen, E., & Brady, S. M. (1990). AIDS risk and prevention for the chronic mentally ill. *Hospital and Community Psychiatry.*

Gordon, G., and T. Klouda. 1989. *Preventing a Crisis: AIDS and Family Planning Work:* London: International Planned Parenthood Federation.

Hope, A.S., Timmel and P. Hodzi. 1984. *Training for Transformation: A Handbook for Community Workers.* Gweru, Zimbabwe: Mambo Press.

Obbo, C., 1993. HIV Transmission Through Social and Geographical Networks in Uganda. *Social Science and Medicine.*

Piette, J. D., Thompson, B. J., Fleishman, J. A., & Mor, V. (1993). The organisation and delivery of AIDS case management.

In V. J. Lynch, G. A. Lloyd, & M. Fimbres (Eds.), *The changing face of AIDS: Implications for social work practice.* Westport, CT: Auburn House.

Schoepf, B.G. 1983. Health for Rural Women. *Community Action* (Zimbabwe).

Sierra Health Foundation (1991). *Challenge for the future: Coordinating HIV/AIDS care and services in the next decade.* Rancho Cordova.

Yates, B., 1982, Colonialism, Education and Work: Sex Differentiation in Colonial Zaire. In: *Women Work in Africa*, edited by E.G. Bay. Boulder, CO: Westview Press.

2

HIV Baby Booms

Worldwide AIDS cannot be explained by a single virus causing a single and continuous epidemic. Instead, worldwide spread is the work of a virus family of types, subtypes and strains that cause more or less related epidemics. Each member of the family has its own distinctive behaviour and each epidemic runs its own distinctive course.

In 1985 Montagnier and Clavel studied a patient from Guinea-Bissau who definitely had AIDS but no HIV antibodies according to available tests. They found in his blood another virus that seemed in many ways related to Western HIV but different enough to be considered a second AIDS virus. It was named HIV-2 and the original HIV was renamed HIV-1 from then on. HIV-2 was subsequently found in all AIDS cases seronegative for HIV-1, that is, virtually all cases seen in West Africa. This was the first evidence that AIDS epidemics could spring from different but related virus types.

Now that we have the laboratory tools to identify them, we can look back on the discovery of three HIV types and behaviours: HIV-1 in 1983, HIV-2 in 1985 and HIV-0 in 1990. They are responsible for at least three distinct AIDS epidemics that affect distinct regions of the world. The HIV-1 epidemic spreads rapidly from widely scattered foci; HIV-2 spreads slowly in West Africa and, recently, more rapidly in India; HIV-0 spreads, just barely, in only one part of Africa. These three viruses differ in their appearance, method of transmission, activity and time and place of occurrence. To trace the movements and virulence of a particular virus, one must be able to recognise that virus with absolute certainty. A nonvisual method is needed because ordinary microscopy sees cells but not viruses. Electron microscopy sees viruses within cells but is unable to recognise and distinguish HIV types.

In 1986 a nonvisual method was discovered by three independent research groups. Two worked in the United States, headed, respectively, by Palker of Duke University and Rusche of Repligen and one worked in the Netherlands (Meloen and Goudsmit). The method is based on a variable signature site in the outer coat of HIV. Whether type 0, 1, or 2, every HIV contains this site. In its variation, this signature serves to identify not only the HIV type but its subtype and strain.

What exactly is this viral signature that tells us so much? Its shell, or capsid, is surrounded by a membrane plus an envelope. The envelope is not a continuous barrier but a network of two inter-locked proteins that protrude from the membrane much as hairs protrude from our skin.

Like all proteins, these envelope proteins consist of amino acids in a particular sequence. In the outermost protein, most of the sequence is fixed, or constant, but a few regions or domains are variable. The so-called third variable domain, or V3, contains the signature site. It is a site to which HIV antibodies respond. When we generate antibodies against invaders of our system, they are keyed to very specific parts of those invaders: to certain proteins or, more accurately, to six to ten amino acids within those proteins. The antibodies are configured to bind to this site.

When we detect antibody configuration, we learn the topography of their binding site. So when we analyse antibodies to the V3 region of a particular HIV, we detect the topography or signature of that site. This tells us the HIV type, subtype and strain. Just one fingerprick of blood from an HIV-infected person (about 10 microliters, or 1/100 of a millilitre) contains one to ten thousand viral particles, which is more than enough for two different methods of signature detection. Antibody analysis, just described, is quick and easy and quite accurate as to virus type.

However, it is somewhat less accurate as to subtype and much less accurate as to strain. So for highest accuracy, virologists use molecular techniques to decipher the nucleic acid coding region for the viral signature, that is, the stretch of nucleic acids that codes for the amino acids at the signature site. For HIV this gene fragment can be found in the DNA of host blood cells at points where HIV has been integrated. Alternatively, it can be found in the cell-free HIV RNA that circulates in the host serum.

The molecular method currently requires twenty-four hours for computerised determination and analysis of the viral signature. The result reliably tells you HIV type 0, 1, or 2 and, just as reliably, the subtype and strain. The computer groups viruses by comparing their coding regions and counting the nucleotides by which they differ.

The quick and easy antibody method is usually sufficient for rough distinctions of type and subtype that reveal broad epidemic patterns. It is used to tell whether HIV-0 or HIV-2 is on the move; whether HIV-1 subtype B or E is spreading in Asia; whether HIV-1B is rising or failing in a particular area or moving from one group to another; whether HIV-1C has travelled from Africa to India. However, only the delicate molecular techniques can reliably reveal viral strains. These can tell us who infected whom and whether Gallo's HIV-1 IIIB is—or is not—the same as Montagnier's HIV-1 Lai. Both of these techniques to detect HIV signatures have vastly improved understanding of the current AIDS epidemics.

These HIVs are not harmless to the humans -they infect. They are eventually lethal but allow a relatively long symptom-free period compared with HIV-1. They maintain a low level of endemicity in limited parts of the world that are probably close to their animal source or reservoir. In this reservoir they remain a harmless cousin of HIV (*i.e.*, SIV), which may help to explain why they are not more lethal in humans. They have not yet had to change much to adapt to their new host. If allowed to spread rapidly in an environment that is new and far from their reservoir, HIV-0 and HIV-2 might well begin to kill us more quickly.

HIV-2 has at least three subtypes (maybe many more), none of which is confined to just one geographic area. HIV-2 subtype A is found in Senegal, the Cape Verde Islands, Mali, Ghana, Gambia and Guinea-Bissau. HIV-2 subtype B is widespread in West Africa. Nowhere is either subtype a great threat to the general population, but since both HIV-2A and HIV-2B circulate in West Africa, they can infect cells of the same individual. This leads to viral sex and recombinant offspring, as are seen in many cases of West African HIV-2 infection.

HIV reproduction requires the active participation of a third party: the living host cell. HIV can enter and infect its favourite immune cell at any time, but the virus is quiescent as long as the cell is quiescent. It cannot do its damage until converted to DNA and integrated into the cell genome. This happens when the resting cell is activated by the threat of some foreign invader. When the immune cell multiplies in response to the invader, HIV enters the cell genome and begins to multiply, using the cellular reproductive machinery.

Most organisms have only one reproductive choice, HIVs have two choices. They can reproduce sexually, by the mating of two parents (our only choice), or they can reproduce asexually (the only choice of most microorganisms). In asexual reproduction, the genes of one generation are copied or cloned to the next. Sexual reproduction can also produce clones, as when a host cell is infected by two identical viruses, that is, HIVs having two identical strands of RNA.

By definition, clones are exact copies, but HIV cloning is careless and produces many inexact copies. This accounts for some of the change we see in the HIV family, though not the remarkable pace or degree of change. It does not explain the successive new waves of HIV that are quite distinct from their parents yet still able to cause AIDS.

Such change is possible only with sexual reproduction and recombination. This requires infection of the host cell by viruses that are not identical but have enough genetic overlap to permit crossover of genetic information. Their mating produces offspring of three kinds. Two are homozygous, that is, one has two identical RNA strands like one parent; the other has two identical RNA strands like the other parent. The third is heterozygous, having one RNA strand from each parent. These heterozygotes look like either parent but have characteristics of both. They do not, themselves, represent remarkable change, but their mating does. When heterozygotes infect a new cell, they produce recombinant offspring. Each virus of this new generation has two identical RNA strands that mix genes of both father and mother. Recombinant offspring are not always better than their parents, but recombination allows variation and flexibility.

In retroviruses like HIV that reproduce quickly and often, recombination allows major change in a short time. It can eliminate mutations from the father or mother that are deleterious to the virus. It can enable rapid adaptation to a new host or mode of transmission. HIVs continually mate and produce recombinant off spring completely new viruses with completely new characteristics—which predicts that AIDS epidemics will continually rise and fall around the world.

GLOBAL SURVEY OF HIV

Many recombinant offspring of HIV-2A and HIV-2B tell us that these two subtypes have long inhabited the same region and population, causing double infections in many individuals. Their confinement, until recently, to very restricted and overlapping areas in West Africa suggests a local source for HIV-2. Only in West Africa are there regions where the majority of AIDS cases are caused by HIV-2. Even in regions where HIV-1 now has the lion's share, HIV-2 keeps a small but steady percentage of all HIV infections. However, its share of AIDS cases is even smaller than its share of HIV infections. Since HIV-2 infections progress to AIDS very slowly or not at all, the great majority (over 95 per cent) of AIDS in West Africa is caused by HIV-1, largely subtype A.

Exposure to HIV-2 leads much less frequently to infection and AIDS than does exposure to HIV-1A. Recent evidence suggests that individuals exposed to both HIV-2 and HIV-1A may gain some benefit from HIV-2. It does not completely protect against infection by HIV-1A, since many individuals show evidence of both infections. But it may slow the rapid disease course of HIV-1A since HIV-2 infects the same type of cell as HIV-1. The fact that they are cross-competitors suggests that these viruses are related and evolved from a distant common ancestor. If so, HIV-1 has evolved much farther from the presumably harmless ancestor because it is now far more harmful than HIV-2. Both HIV-2 and HIV-1A are typically transmitted by heterosexual (*i.e.*, vaginal) intercourse, but HIV-2 seems ill adapted to this route.

It rarely establishes a new infection and when it does, the infection is low-grade, resulting in a slow and sometimes inapparent disease course. In a low-grade infection, diagnosis is possible but isolation of the virus is difficult. The HIV-2 virus load is small and causes only short periods of acute illness. Individuals infected with HIV-2 rarely develop AIDS. This picture of low infectivity and slow disease course will probably remain as long as the opportunity to transmit HIV-2 remains low. The opportunity is unlikely to change in West Africa and, when HIV-2 appears in Europe and Asia, it so far appears in West African immigrants or their partners. If HIV-2 remains thus limited to its accustomed place and people, it may never take off. But the history of HIV-1 warns against complacency.

Since HIV-2 spreads poorly by heterosexual relations, it may spread better by homosexual relations. If so, one fears that HIV-2 is potentially as dangerous as HIV-1. It simply has not yet bumped into the population that can spread it rapidly. We have seen that rapid circulation alone can start a chain reaction of HIV infections that progress faster and more frequently to AIDS. If HIV-2A is now spreading heterosexually among prostitutes in India, this scenario may already be under way.

The story of HIV-0 is in many respects very similar to the story of HIV-2. In 1990, in a couple from Cameroon, van der Groen and not found HIV strains highly divergent from HIV-1 and HIV-2. Several other research teams subsequently isolated similar strains from other AIDS patients, all from Cameroon or Gabon. Many of these patients showed no HIV-1 or HIV-2 antibodies in response to the customary HIV tests. They were infected with strains now designated HIV-0, which infects almost exclusively people living in Cameroon and Gabon.

The virus has been found in Europe but, as with HIV-2, it has been found only in immigrants from its source countries or in their sex partners. Even in Cameroon and Gabon, HIV-0 infections are extremely rare. Among HIV-positive individuals in those areas, the culprit is usually HIV-1A and this is even more the case among those who have AIDS. The situation echoes HIV-2 versus HIV-1A in West Africa. At this point about twenty HIV-0 strains have been isolated. Study of their signature V3 sequences suggests that this virus is at least as variable as HIV- 1. But whereas HIV-1 subtypes tend to have diverse habitats, HIV-0 strains share the same or overlapping habitats. Their distinguishing features are as yet unclear, either because data are lacking or because their differentiation is incomplete.

Distinct HIV subtypes are believed to form through competition and adaptation to various hosts. HIV-0 lacks subtypes because it has not yet faced these challenges. HIV-0 infections have so far occurred only after heterosexual transmission. They are far less widespread than infections with HIV-1 A or any other heterosexually transmitted HIV-1 subtypes. But as with HIV-2, this does not mean HIV-0 could not become a killer under the right circumstances. At this point, we may see HIV-0 and HIV-2 stalled or suspended at a stage that HIV-1 left decades ago. HIV-1 has moved on and now rarely behaves like HIV-2. For HIV-2, the picture is reversed: it rarely behaves like the more virulent HIV-1. Sparse data on HIV-0 keep us guessing about its strength.

However, like HIV-2, it has not reached high infectivity and therefore, though ultimately fatal, it does not threaten to become stronger and more widespread in its home area. Both HIV-2 and HIV-0 remain confined and unrelated to the mainstream AIDS epidemic, but they could soar, given the chance. Clearly AIDS can be caused by more than one HIV type, though HIV-1 is currently the main killer. HIV-1B dominates in Europe and the United States, while HIV-1A is more common in Africa. Are these the only HIV-1 subtypes? Are they the same or similar in their level of infectivity, virulence and mode of transmission? As might be expected from our comparison of HIV-0, HIV-1 and HIV-2, the answer is a resounding no. Eight subtypes of HIV-1 have already been identified.

Apparently, once a HIV-1 subtype is established in a geographic niche, other HIV-1 subtypes have difficulty penetrating that area. This is the net effect of what may be considered a viral war. Multiple HIV-1 subtypes may move into a certain population, but depending on their infectivity or transmission characteristics, one subtype will pull ahead in the competition. It survives and wins the niche because, by definition, it is the fittest: it spreads most efficiently in the population.

More rarely, two or more subtypes with equal advantages will end up sharing a population. However, win or draw, the viral war goes on. Peace is only temporary because stronger and more aggressive subtypes keep turning up. No matter how perfectly subtypes are adapted to their hosts, they can always be displaced by changes in the population (*e.g.*, in sexual practices) or changes in competing subtypes.

At any moment, the formerly fittest subtype can be overtaken by one even more fit. A niche holder may lose its hold, especially if recombination suddenly produces a subtype with markedly superior advantages. These notions point to subtype-specific AIDS epidemics that are separate and distinct in time, location and other features. Their agents are separate and distinct in transmission route, infectivity and aggressivity. They do not merge despite continual strain variation within subtypes.

Since the beginning of the AIDS epidemic in Amsterdam, we have studied more than a hundred HIV-1B strains in newly infected individuals. What we observed was quite remarkable. As expected, strain variation accumulated as the epidemic progressed and involved more individuals. However, over these ten to twelve years of viral replication, the strains remained recognisable as members of subtype B. They infected thousands of new hosts and went through millions of replication cycles.

Each replication yielded mutation of at least one of the 10,000 nucleic acids of the AIDS virus genome. But the virus infecting people in 1990 looked surprisingly similar to the virus infecting people in 1980. This stability strongly suggests that early in an epidemic, a particular AIDS virus adapts rapidly to its host. It evolves optimal reproduction characteristics for a particular method of virus dissemination. Subsequently, all strains of the virus population conserve the genetic characteristics that have guaranteed the success of their subtype. That is, the strains with these characteristics thrive while those without them disappear.

Some HIV-1 subtypes occupy very large territories; others rule small areas. There is good reason to believe that, whatever their realm, the subtype-specific epidemics are prone to change at any time. A subtype can even die out, if only because its most infectious strains die with their victims. In fact, we see evidence that the HIV-1B epidemic has peaked in the West. In the United States and Europe, it seems to be fading, at least from its primary risk groups of gay men and drug users. The number of new HIV-1B infections in these groups has stopped rising and may even be declining, especially in Western Europe. It looks as if the first major HIV-1B epidemic has completed its natural cycle of logarithmic increase and has begun its retreat.

HIV-1B may well have been endemic in Europe long before the American outbreak of the early 1980s. With a low level of infectivity and aggressivity, it resembled today's HIV-2 (lethal but slow) or the Jembrana virus of cattle (not always lethal). It rarely caused disease following heterosexual transmission or blood transmission. However, once it entered the emancipated gay community, it adapted to invade humans through the inner walls of the rectum. Rapid circulation allowed it to become the efficient killer we see today.

In the United States, for the first ten to fifteen years of the epidemic, about 50 per cent of all AIDS cases occurred among gay men. In Europe the percentage was smaller, but only because it combined the very low percentage of gay AIDS cases in southern Europe (where AIDS is seen mainly in IV drug users) with the very high per cent in northern Europe. In northern cities like Amsterdam, 75 per cent of AIDS cases still occur in the gay community.

HIV-1B may be fading slightly among gay men and IV drug users, but this does not mean that AIDS will vanish from the Western world. Subtypes could be imported that excel HIV-1B in their rate of heterosexual transmission. Studies in Thailand show that HIV-1E has a 75 per cent chance of heterosexual transmission, whereas HIV-1B has a 25 per cent chance. In other words, of one hundred people exposed to HIV-1E by heterosexual relations, seventy-five are likely to be infected; with HIV-1B, twenty-five are likely to be infected. For HIV-1B to cause a heterosexual epidemic, a homosexual or anal factor seems to be required. In Haiti, for example, HIV was probably introduced by gay tourists from the United States who sought sex with young male prostitutes. The Haitian men they infected with HIV-1B then infected wives and girlfriends, particularly since heterosexual couples in Latin America commonly use anal sex as a no-cost contraceptive measure.

In most of the United States and Western Europe, other contraceptive measures are generally affordable and preferred. For this and other cultural reasons, anal sex is less popular among heterosexual couples in these regions, so their risk of HIV-1B infection remains relatively low. But if not displaced by a more efficient subtype, HIV-1B could change. It could come to rely less on anal transmission and more on vaginal transmission. Some data suggest that because certain cells are more abundant in vaginal than rectal tissue, the HIVs best at vaginal transmission are those best at entering these cells. HIV-1B strains with this knack could someday appear and gradually outcompete HIV-1B strains limited to anal transmission.

As always, this would be a random process, not the result of a viral conspiracy! Natural selection simply favours the preservation and accumulation of accidental changes that prove to be advantageous. In this case, strains with the knack would simply survive better than those without it.

A fierce debate rages as to whether HIV-1B has already begun to change. There is strong concern that it is shifting from the population of gay men and IV drug users to the general population, especially women. The percentage of US women among AIDS patients has indeed risen since 1985—even doubled, according to some data. However, a similar rise has not been seen in Europe and we lack hard evidence that HIV-1B has actually become more efficient in spreading to women. Three factors help to explain this apparent contradiction.

First of all, as gay men decrease their share of total AIDS cases, women's share increases even if their actual number of cases remains the same. Second, some US women who are counted as AIDS patients have HIV infection combined with female diseases like cervical cancer. These diseases or their treatment can aggravate HIV infection and hasten development of AIDS. They do not themselves cause immunodeficiency but, since 1993, women with such diseases have been defined as AIDS patients when HIV infection is also present. Finally, if HIV-1B actually infects more US women, they are primarily women of a certain behavioural group, not women in general. They are poor black and Hispanic women of US inner cities, but their AIDS risk is only marginally tied to poverty, race or sex with an HIV-positive partner. It is mainly tied to drug use.

In New York, for example, two-thirds of the black and Hispanic women with AIDS are IV drug users. Of the rest, most have sex with a drug user. If a poor black or Hispanic woman lives in a community at high risk for AIDS but avoids drug use and sex with drug users, her chance of infection is negligible. It thus appears that HIV-1B has not actually or appreciably improved its rate of hetero-sexual transmission.

The virus is bound to move from the gay to the general population, especially in urban centers. How much and how fast this happens varies from city to city depending, in each locale, on the distance and interface between the gay population and the drug-using population of the inner city. Still, heterosexual transmission per se seems to have little impact on the inner-city spread of HIV. Except among IV drug users, such transmission remains rare unless assisted by special circumstances: preexisting venereal disease, or unusually high virus load in the male partner or anal intercourse. Studies in Thailand showed that even frequency of intercourse did not promote the transmission of HIV-1B as long as the intercourse was vaginal, not anal.

Thailand is the main focus of HIV-1B in Southeast Asia. The virus has also been exported to South America, mainly Brazil. In Thailand it first surfaced in 1987 among IV drug users in the southern capital city of Bangkok. So HIV-1 subtype B had apparently spread from Europe to the United States and Haiti, then to Thailand. It is not far-fetched to assume that its spread was related to sex tourism followed by dissemination in the Thai IV drug-using population. Thailand may have no more prostitution than other Asian countries, but its commercial sex industry is more socially and officially accepted. Younger and younger women are working as prostitutes because they can be promoted as virgins, free of HIV. They are often recruited from remote villages to ensure minimal exposure to sex or disease. A convenient myth circulates that young girls, even nonvirgins, are somehow impervious to HIV. To its credit, Thailand has now begun to work hard on HIV-related problems.

In 1989 a second HIV-1 epidemic emerged in the north of Thailand, but the agent was subtype E. Rarely seen before, HIV-1E rapidly spread south by heterosexual transmission, invading the territory of subtype B: the IV drug users. Today subtype B is becoming scarce throughout

Thailand and is not spreading to the rest of Asia. This again proves that HIV-1B is well adapted to spread and do harm through anal sexual intercourse but ill adapted to do harm through vaginal intercourse. It competes poorly with subtypes more efficient in heterosexual transmission.

In West Africa and other parts of Africa, HIV-1A is the dominant AIDS-causing virus. Spread easily through heterosexual intercourse, it is overtaking the slow but steady HIV-2 and is competing with HIV-1D for dominance in central Africa. Whether 1A or 1D will win is unclear. Already we see recombinants of A and D viruses, so the victory may go to descendants with the best characteristics of both. Wherever they occur, recombination events sustain HIV and AIDS by adding new viruses to the circulating mix. Recently, a study of Rwandan women documented the emergence of an HIV-1A/C recombinant that is already capable of infection and transmission to a new host.

HIV-1A has not spread to Asia, but its genes have. The emerging threat to Asians, HIV-1E, is actually a recombinant virus that inherited all its genes from HIV-1A, except the one that codes for the viral envelope. That gene comes from its other parent. The recombination event probably occurred in central Africa since both HIV-1A and the recombinant 1E are found there. Remarkably, the parent that contributed the envelope gene has not yet been found anywhere. It is very rare or even extinct, suggesting that the recombination event must have occurred long ago. The fact that HIV-1E spreads much better in Asia than in Africa points strongly to host or genetic factors. Apparently, the cells of Asians are more susceptible to 1E infection than to 1A infection and, conversely, the cells of Africans are more susceptible to 1A than 1E.

The theory is that central African drug smugglers, infected with HIV-1E, brought the virus to Thailand. The virus is so infectious through heterosexual intercourse that it is now spreading in all of Asia with devastating effects. In its rapid journey through Asia, it has learned to spread very fast in a dense population. If we could stop only one AIDS virus, it should be this one, since it threatens by far the largest concentration of people.

The only other AIDS virus now on the rise is HIV-1 subtype C. This virus was first documented among the populations of Ethiopia and Somalia. It then moved south to South Africa and its neighbours and from there to India by a path similar to that followed by HIV-2A. HIV-1C recently emerged in Central America and has also reached China. In the spread of various subtypes, China is an important and special case. At first, all reported cases were HIV-1B. They occurred in Yunnan Province, which has points of contact with Vietnam, Laos, Thailand and Myanmar (Burma). But the virus was actually a Thai variant, known as HIV-1B', which probably entered China with infected drug users or dealers crossing the Yunnan border.

At the same time, Chinese women who had worked in Thailand as prostitutes came back infected with HIV-1E. But since 1990, most strains found among infected drug users of Yunnan are HIV-1C. Not found in Thailand, this subtype has apparently come to China from some other area, so far unknown. A viral war between subtypes C and E seems imminent in this part of the world.

AIDS is not caused by a single virus but by very different viruses from one big HIV family. Each one of the family can cause AIDS but at various rates—an important distinguishing feature. Some have acquired the characteristic to be infectious primarily through entry in the gut of men and women (*i.e.*, the anal mucosa of the lower intestine), while others are more infectious through entry in the vagina (or the penis, though this is relatively rare). Some of these viruses, like HIV-0 and HIV-2, are endemic in very small regions of the world. They have not yet caused large-scale AIDS epidemics, mainly because they have not encountered the right opportunity. HIV-1B had the opportunity and caused a large epidemic that now seems to be winding down. Meanwhile, others are on the rise, threatening epidemics of immense proportions: HIV-1E and C in Asia; HIV-1A and D in Africa. We see no indication that HIV-1 subtypes are merging into one supersubtype.

And in the course of an epidemic, though variation accumulates within the responsible subtype, every new strain looks very much like those that infected people at the beginning of that epidemic. However, we see that one subtype can overtake another, as is now happening in Thailand.

When a subtype is battling another for dominance, the losing virus has only one chance for survival. It can pass its genes to the conquering virus through recombination. Viruses of the HIV family continually interbreed to perpetuate the family trade, even at the cost of an individual virus subtype or strain. Viral sex allows variation while preserving the unique genetic characteristics of the family: the ability to replicate and spread through cells of the immune system of the host. All members of the family infect a host by entering CD_4^+ immune cells, where they replicate. The offspring burst from the cells into extracellular fluid, by which they are transmitted (by sexual relations or exchange of blood) to a new host and breeding ground.

Or before they burst out, the virus particles are transmitted within the infected cell and are disgorged in the new host. Either way, the old host is then useless and the parent viruses are headed for extinction. Their fate does not matter, now that the offspring have found a new host. However, the moribund parent viruses continue to circulate, eventually causing AIDS and killing the discarded host. HIV types and subtypes can be considered distinct viruses since they remain stable while accommodating enormous strain variation. Even if they share a common ancestor, their distribution history will vary, depending on many circumstances.

As an example, we can look at the history of HIV-1B in Thailand. The virus surfaced in 1987 and within a year had started an AIDS epidemic among drug users in Bangkok. In one to two years, it was spreading from drug users to male and female prostitutes and their clients, particularly soldiers. The virus circulating among drug users seemed to be the same virus circulating sexually, but this was not quite true. By the early 1990s, the virus of Bangkok drug users belonged to the HIV-1B subtype and probably came from the West.

However, a close look found genetic differences that put it in a new category. Now called HIV-1B, it is similar to HIV-1B but very distinct from HIV-1E, the subgroup spreading rapidly in Thailand and the rest of Asia. Initially, the E virus was found largely in cases of sexual transmission, not transmission by drug use. HIV-1E infected very few drug users in the late 1980s but is now overtaking both HIV-1B and HIV-1B' in that risk group.

Researchers at the Centers for Disease Control in Atlanta have recently traced the history of HIV-1B, HIV-1B' and HIV-1E in Thailand, mainly by looking at two groups of Thai prison inmates. The first group included ten drug users infected with HIV-1B in 1986 and 1987, before the Thai epidemic took off. The second included three men who were infected once the epidemic was in full swing: one by HIV-1E and two by HIV-1B. In the first group the ten infecting strains were indistinguishable from those circulating in Europe and the United States. They were true HIV-1 subtype B and even had the same signature in the V3 region as Euro-American strains, which strongly suggests that they were imported by Euro-American travellers.

The ten early-infected men left prison in 1988. They were then free to spread HIV-1B in the drug-using community, but the virus did not thrive. In the West it had been passaged to greater virulence by homosexual intercourse before it entered the drug-using population. This did not happen in Thailand to any great extent. In the West it had no competitors, but in Thailand it faced HIV-1E and HIV-1B. After 1988, HIV-1B was edged out by HIV-1B among drug users, while HIV-1 subtype E spread simultaneously among prostitutes through heterosexual intercourse. Now HIV-1B, is also fading from drug users, edged out by HIV-1E. Clearly, a given HIV virus can be readily replaced—in only a few years—by an HIV better suited for spread in a particular population.

A population may be defined by many factors, ranging from behaviour to racial or ethnic group. Just as HIV-1B and HIV-1B' are less successful than HIV-1B in a heterosexual population, they may also be less successful among certain Asian peoples. As individuals worldwide vary in their strengths and weaknesses-including their susceptibility to this or that disease—so do ethnic groups. They are, after all, collections of individuals who share a common background and physiology, however diluted by time and distance. All other things being equal, host factors make a difference. Many diseases vary in prevalence from Caucasians to Africans to Asians.

Many occur in just one subgroup that has special susceptibility. For example, Tay-Sachs disease occurs almost exclusively among northeast European Jews or their descendants, regardless of where those descendants live today. The rarity of HIV-1B among Africans suggests that they resist it better than do Euro-Americans. Perhaps Asians also resist HIV-1B while being, like Africans, easy prey to other subtypes.

OUTGROWTH OF SUBTYPES

If they are truly different viruses, their worldwide spread is directed by chance within transmissibility limits, since subtypes are not equally well spread by anal or vaginal intercourse. This seems indicated by a small study we performed in Russia, Byelorussia and Lithuania. The viruses we studied in the former Soviet Union did not cluster geographically but according to risk groups based on behaviour. Thus, of seven HIV-infected people who had acquired the virus by homosexual intercourse, all seven were infected by HIV-1B, whether they lived in Vilnius, Lithuania, or Moscow.

Of six heterosexually infected people, all six had HIV-1C, whether residents of Minsk, Byelorussia, or Rostov in Russia. Perhaps most ominous, four people infected through drug use in various cities had four different types: HIV-1A, C, D and G. Apparently, any subtype passes with ease among drug users, whether it is suited to anal or vaginal transmission. If so, drug use is the best and perhaps the main vehicle for a subtype to enter a new area. However, once introduced, a new subtype may fail to thrive, as HIV-1B has so far failed in Thailand.

That the HIV-1 subtypes were truly separate well before the 1980s can be extrapolated from the genetic history of HIV-1A and 1B, the two we know best. HIV-1A was first isolated from a sample taken in Tanzania in 1976. Allowing for strain variation, that virus is indistinguishable from today's HIV-1A viruses, so the origin of the subtypes must lie before 1976 and, more specifically, before the AIDS epidemic became apparent.

Subtype emergence most likely resulted from the successful adaptation of HIV to spread in the human population. The same can be said for HIV-1B. The viruses isolated from individuals infected in Amsterdam in the early 1980s are not markedly different from those found in people infected ten years later. The genetic data on HIV-1A and 1B indicate that neither is the ancestor of the other. Also, HIV-1 subtypes are relatively stable on a gene-by-gene basis.

Point mutations of genes result in proliferation of strains within a subtype, but strains do not leave the subtype or merge with other strains. Some subtypes show, more strain variation than others, so either their evolution is faster or they are older. In any case, subtypes must be independent entities that predate the epidemic status of HIV (though not necessarily its ability to cause immune deficiency). For at least two decades—millions of generations for HIV—the subtypes have been genetically stable entities in which point mutations can occur without loss of basic characteristics defining the subtype.

If the HIV-0, HIV-1 and HIV-2 types and subtypes predate any AIDS epidemic, where did they originate? As to HIV-0 and HIV-2, the answer is relatively easy. They have so far caused only small outbreaks of AIDS in Africa. Their appearance on other continents has been traced directly back to Africa. So they originated in Africa. The same is less clear-cut but appears to be true for the HIV-1 subtypes. All those known to us can be found somewhere in Africa even if, like HIV-1B, they are very rare on that continent. More important, multiple HIV-1 subtypes have cocirculated in several parts of Africa and, until very recently, on no other continent. Since cocirculation of subtypes is necessary for creation of new subtypes, Africa was the first place this process could occur, as far as we know.

New subtypes result when two nonidentical parent subtypes infect a single host cell. If they produce a recombinant virus particularly fit for survival in a particular population, it may become a viable new and even dominant subtype, such as HIV-1E in Asia. The chance for such success depends on the level at which subtypes cocirculate and on the frequency of new infections. As one or both rise, the resulting rise in recombinants—in sheer number and genetic variety—increases the potential for new subtypes. About 10 per cent of worldwide HIV-1 viruses can be earmarked as recombinants of HIV-1 subtypes. All HIV-1 subtypes have participated in recombination, as have all HIV-2 subtypes. But HIV-1 and HIV-2 subtypes mix only among themselves, not with each other. HIV-1 subtypes are sexually incompatible with HIV-2 subtypes.

Like humans and chimpanzees, they are closely related but cannot mate and produce a hybrid. Whether HIV-0 viruses can mate and produce recombinants with HIV-1 or HIV-2 viruses is unlikely and so far not described despite the recent description of individuals coinfected with HIV-0 and HIV-1. That is the main reason to use the term HIV-0, unlike those researchers who group HIV-0 viruses with HIV-1 as "subtype 0".

These six parent subtypes must have emerged previously from dramatic events, such as cross-species transmissions, in Africa. After passing from their animal reservoir to humans, these progenitor subtypes pursued their independent ways, adapting to new environments and spawning variants. Such far-reaching development is plausible because their histories span several decades.

SELECTED READINGS

Boyd-Franklin, N., Steiner, G. L., & Boland, M. G. (Eds.) (1995). *Children, Families and HIV/AIDS*. New York: Guildford Press.

Levine, C., & Stein, G. (1994). Orphans *of the HIV epidemic.* New York: The Orphan Project.

Oaklander, V. (1998). *Windows to our children.* Highland, NY: Center for Gestalt Development.

Tross, S., & Hirsch, S. (1988). Psychological distress and neuropsychological complications of HIV infection and AIDS. *American Psychologist.*

Ward-Wimmer, D., and Riley, M. (1991). *Caring at home.* Washington, DC: Child Welfare League of America.

3

Epidemiology of HIV

Most of the variation in trajectories of the HIV/AIDS epidemic across world regions can be explained by differences in behaviour across societies and across groups within societies, which are in turn influenced by many of the economic and cultural factors. In the absence of a cure or a vaccine, the key to arresting the spread of HIV is changing behaviour.

The epidemiology of HIV/AIDS suggests two important objectives for public programs to slow the spread of HIV: governments should act as soon as possible and, irrespective of the stage of the epidemic, they should ensure prevention of infection among those with the riskiest. The extent to which HIV has saturated subpopulations with high-risk behaviour and spread outward to those with low-risk behaviour has important implications for government priorities in preventing HIV.

The rate of spread of HIV and current levels of infection are measured by incidence and prevalence.

— The incidence of HIV is the number of new cases, that is, the number of people who become infected during a specified period of time, usually over a twelve-month interval.

— The prevalence of HIV is the number of people currently infected with HIV at a given point in time. Because there is no cure for HIV/AIDS, HIV prevalence reflects the cumulative numbers of infections from the past and the mortality rate of those infected.

At the beginning of the epidemic, HIV prevalence grows rapidly and AIDS mortality is not yet evident because of the long asymptomatic period of most of those infected. Years later, when the first cases of AIDS appear, large numbers of people are already infected with HIV. Incidence may still be climbing but growth in prevalence may slow because of rising HIV/AIDS mortality or saturation of the population. As long as incidence exceeds mortality, the prevalence of HIV will continue to rise.

Prevalence will peak in the year in which incidence exactly equals the rising mortality rate. Whether prevalence then levels off, declines, or resumes climbing toward a new peak will depend on whether the number of new infections is equal to, less than, or greater than the number of deaths of people with HIV/AIDS. In the absence of a cure, the key to reducing future HIV prevalence is by preventing new cases—that is, lowering incidence. Stable or declining prevalence does not necessarily signal the end of the epidemic.

Eventually, HIV prevalence will level off in all populations; in some it will stabilise at a high level and in others at a low level. The factors affecting the height of the plateau in HIV prevalence are discussed below. However, a plateau simply indicates that there is an equilibrium in which the number of new infections exactly offsets AIDS mortality. In populations where prevalence is declining, mortality is occurring at a faster rate than new infections. The number of new infections may still be quite high, coexisting with high mortality. The relationship between HIV incidence and prevalence and the lag in the appearance of AIDS cases have important implications for public policy:

— Early intervention is critical to prevent an AIDS epidemic that can persist for decades. Only a fraction of those infected with HIV are showing symptoms of AIDS at any given point in time. By the time that AIDS morbidity becomes a significant health issue, HIV may have spread widely in the population, making prevention efforts very difficult. Countries with few reported AIDS cases should not be complacent about launching prevention campaigns.

— The full impact of infection levels on mortality is delayed. Even if all new HIV infections could be prevented, in the absence of a cure, AIDS deaths would continue for years because of the population already infected and the long asymptomatic period between HIV infection and AIDS. Countries where HIV prevalence is high are only beginning to experience the profound mortality impact of the epidemic, which will last for decades even with the best prevention efforts.

BIOLOGY AND BEHAVIOUR

The reproductive rate of a sexually transmitted disease is the average number of susceptible people infected by an infected person over his or her lifetime.

If each person infected with a disease transmits it to exactly one other person, then the reproductive rate is 1. In populations in which HIV has a reproductive rate of less than 1, the epidemic will not be self-sustaining. Thus, the greater the reproductive rate of HIV, the more rapidly the epidemic will spread.

The most common mode of transmission of HIV is through sexual contact. Three main factors have a large influence on the reproductive rate of all sexually transmitted diseases (STDs), including HIV:

— the amount of time a person remains infectious
— the risk of transmission per sexual contact
— the rate of acquisition of new partners.

These factors are similar for transmission through contaminated injecting equipment, except that the risk of transmission per contact refers to the risk per injection and the number of partners refers to number of people with whom injecting equipment is shared. The broad points in the following discussion therefore apply to transmission through sharing of contaminated needles, as well as through sexual contact. Each of these three factors is in turn influenced by the biology of the virus and by individual behaviour.

Biology plays an important role in the amount of time a

person remains infectious and in the risk of transmission per contact. But individual behaviour also has a strong influence on the risk of transmission per contact—for example, through decisions on condom use, disinfecting shared needles and seeking treatment for other STDs. And individual behaviour has a direct relation with the rate of partner acquisition. Until medical science discovers either a cure vaccine, the most important avenue for reducing the spread of HIV will continue to be changing individual behaviour.

Duration of infectiousness

The long duration of HIV infectiousness increases the likelihood that an infected individual will pass the infection to others. Further, because a person with HIV typically remains asymptomatic for years, an infected individual and his or her sexual (or injecting) partners are often unaware of the risk of transmission. Thus, the long duration of asymptomatic HIV infection potentially puts many more partners at risk than is the case for other STDs. The impact of recently developed drugs that extend the lives of people with HIV may lengthen the infectious period.

However, if these drugs significantly reduce the viral load, they might reduce the risk of infection per contact. Be that as it may, unless both dramatic medical advances and significant reductions in the costs occur, these new drugs are unlikely to have a significant impact on the duration of infectiousness in developing countries, since few developing countries have the financial or human resources to provide them. That leaves two primary mechanisms for prevention—reductions in the risk of infection per contact and reductions in the acquisition of new partners.

The average risk of infection with HIV per sexual exposure is much smaller than that for other sexually transmitted diseases; however, because of the long period of infectiousness and numerous co-factors that enhance HIV transmission, the chance that an HIV-positive person who does not take precautions will eventually infect other can be quite high. The most extensive studies of the risk of HIV transmission per exposure have been conducted in industrial countries. Because of generally superior health levels and the ready availability of treatment for other STDs, the average risk of HIV infection per sexual contact in industrial countries is quite small.

For example, the average chance that an infected male will sexually transmit HIV to an uninfected female partner by unprotected vaginal sex is estimated at between 1 and 2 per cent 1,000 exposures. The risk of transmission from an infected female to an uninfected male partner through unprotected vaginal sex is one-third to one-half as great. Thus, women are believed to have a somewhat greater probability of becoming infected from an infected male partner than the reverse. Anal sex carries the highest risk, especially for the receptive partner. The risk of transmission in unprotected anal intercourse, based on a study of men, is estimated to be between 5 and 30 per cent 1,000 exposures for the receptive partner. However, all of these very likely underestimate—perhaps severely—the average transmission probability per sexual act. They are generally based on studies of transmission within discordant couples—couples in which one partner is HIV-positive and the other is HIV-negative.

Couples that are discordant for a very brief period are not captured in these samples; thus, the most infectious individuals are likely to be excluded. These studies also fail to capture couples in which neither partner tests positive for HIV, but one recently has become infected. A transmission rate per partnership, not taking into account the length of partnership, might be a more realistic measure of the risks of sexual transmission of HIV within relationships. A review of studies of per-partner transmission rates among heterosexuals in the United States and Western Europe found an average transmission probability of about 23 per cent from men to women and of about half that rate (12 per cent) from women to men. The "per contact" risk of HIV transmission with a commercial or casual partner in developing countries is thus likely to be substantially higher.

Notwithstanding these considerations, the average infectiousness of HIV is believed to be substantially less than that for other STDs. Although sexual intercourse is the primary means of HIV transmission in both developed and developing countries, other modes of transmission carry a higher probability of spreading the infection. The chance that a mother will transmit the virus to her infant is variously estimated at 13 to 48 per cent. Transmission probabilities through sharing contaminated injecting equipment between infected and uninfected injecting drug users are variable, depending on the specific injecting practices and which equipment is shared. The probability of transmission through an accidental needle stick in a medical setting, when the needle has been exposed to HIV-infected blood, is only about 1 in 250, or 0.3 per cent. The transmission rate for transfusion of contaminated blood is nearly 100 per cent. The risk of infection per contact is not a constant; it can be influenced by a variety of factors, some of which may tend to exacerbate the epidemic.

Recent studies suggest that infectivity can vary dramatically according to the stage of HIV infection. The two peaks of infectivity are thought to coincide with the periods of highest viral load—the first and highest within the first few months of infection (before the production of antibodies to the virus) and the second, which is thought to be lower, at the very end of the asymptomatic period, as the body loses its battle with HIV. Studies of homosexual men suggest that an individual faces a 10 to 30 per cent chance of becoming infected during a single act of unprotected receptive anal intercourse if his partner is at the early, acute stage of the infection. In the middle stage, the likelihood of infection drops to between 0.01 and 0.1 per cent, but at the end stage it rises again to between 0.1 and 1.0 per cent. The variation in probability of heterosexual transmission in early and late periods of infection has not been estimated but could have important implications for the size of the epidemic.

The likelihood of HIV transmission also differs by the type of the virus. HIV-1 is more easily transmitted and has a shorter incubation period than HIV-2. HIV-1 has many subtypes with specific geographic distributions. However, there is no conclusive epidemiological evidence to date that any of these subtypes are more or less infective than others.

Untreated STDs raise the risk of HIV infection per sexual exposure: STDs are far more common in developing countries than in industrial countries. Studies in both industrial and developing countries have found that people with current or past STDs are 2 to 9 times more likely to be infected with HIV. However, because HIV and other STDs are both highly correlated with risky sexual behaviour—high rates of partner change in particular—it is difficult to disentangle the extent to which conventional STDs actually enhance the transmission of HIV. Nonetheless, there are compelling biological reasons for believing that untreated ulcerative STDs such as herpes, syphilis and chancroid greatly increase the risk of HIV transmission per exposure: the lesions caused by these diseases provide a ready portal for transmission of HIV, whether they are on the HIV-infected or the uninfected partner. Enhanced HIV transmission in the presence of nonulcerative STDs such as gonorrhoea, chlamydia, or trichomoniasis is also biologically plausible but the epidemiological evidence to support it has been weaker, mainly for methodological reasons.

In the early 1990s a randomised controlled trial in rural areas of Mwanza region, Tanzania, found that treatment of symptomatic classic STDs lowered the incidence of HIV among adults by more than 40 per cent. The extent to which this result can he generalised to other countries is likely to depend on many country specific factors, including the underlying prevalence of HIV and STDs, the types of STDs that are prevalent, the quality of treatment services and existing levels of STD treatment prior to the intervention. At the outset of the Mwanza study, HIV prevalence among adults 15 to 54 was already high at 4 per cent. Simulations of the HIV epidemic in rural Uganda indicate that the proportion of HIV infections for which STDs were a cofactor was highest early in that epidemic. This suggests that the effectiveness of STD treatment in slowing HIV incidence in Mwanza might have been even greater had it occurred much earlier in the epidemic.

Male circumcision may be a factor: Some researchers have found a correlation between HIV infection and lack of circumcision and believe that this may account in part for the rapid spread of HIV in sub-Saharan Africa. Ethnographic studies suggest that men are least likely to be circumcised in central, eastern and southern Africa, along a north-south swath through the Rift Valley. This also happens to be the area with the highest rates of HIV infection in urban areas.

One reason why uncircumcised men could be at higher risk of contracting HIV and passing it to others is that they are at higher risk of developing ulcerative STDs, particularly chancroid. Poorer genital hygiene among uncircumcised men may also play a role, particularly in low-income and unsanitary settings.

A study in Kenya found that, even among men without chancroid, uncircumcised men were more likely to sero-convert (29 per cent) than those who were circumcised (2.5 per cent). However, the amount of increased risk of HIV infection from lack of circumcision alone has not been established and whether or not such a risk exists is still debated. This is because circumcision is highly correlated with many other factors besides chancroid.

In particular, ethnicity and religion are strong determinants of whether or not men are circumcised. It is therefore difficult to disentangle the effect of male circumcision (or lack of it) from that of other cultural norms that affect sexual behaviour. Clearly, even if male circumcision is protective against acquiring and spreading HIV, it is not sufficient to prevent infection. High proportions of men in West Africa are circumcised, yet HIV has nonetheless spread rapidly there.

Behaviour affects the probability of transmission. Although the basic transmission probabilities for HIV per exposure are founded in the biology of the virus, fortunately they can be substantially reduced through behavioural change. Using latex condoms and obtaining treatment for conventional STDs can lower the probability of transmission through sexual contact. Sterilisation of injection equipment can dramatically reduce transmission among injecting drug users and among patients in medical facilities.

Rate of partner change

While transmission probabilities have an important influence on the reproductive rate of HIV, the rate of sexual partner change probably accounts for the greatest differences in the rate across groups and countries. Similarly, the rate at which injecting drug users change partners with whom they share unsterilised injecting equipment strongly influences the HIV reproductive rate among them. Finally, in medical settings, the rate of reuse of unsterilised injecting equipment for multiple patients is analytically equivalent to the rate of partner change.

In all three situations, the higher the rate of partner change is, the greater is the likelihood that the virus will pass from infected to uninfected people. In contrast, although the probability of becoming infected per exposure is higher for people receiving transfusions of infected blood and for the children of HIV-positive mothers, these groups are unlikely to infect many others.

Because the HIV reproductive rate for these modes of transmission is probably less than 1, if the virus were spread only by transfusion or from mother to child, the epidemic would most likely not be sustained. In the absence of condom use or sterilisation of shared injecting equipment, rapid rates of partner change sustain the epidemic. Both the average rate of partner change in a population and the variation of the rate across individuals have an impact on the spread of HIV in populations. Other factors being constant, the higher the average rate of partner change is, the higher is the reproductive rate of HIV.

However, in a population in which a few people have very high rates of partner change and many people have very low rates, HIV and other STDs will spread more quickly than if the same average number of partners were distributed more equally across the entire population. Surveys of sexual behaviour suggest that there is in fact quite significant variation in the rate of partner change across subgroups in a single population.

Mixing patterns: The path of the epidemic within the overall population depends on the degree and pattern of mixing among people with high-risk behaviour and the mixing between people with high-risk behaviour and people with low-risk behaviour. By "high-risk behaviour," we mean unprotected sexual intercourse with multiple partners or sharing of unsterilised injecting equipment. People with high-risk behaviour are very likely to become infected and to unknowingly pass HIV to others.

People with low-risk behaviour—who have few partners, who consistently use condoms, who do not inject drugs, or (if they do) do not share injecting equipment—are less likely to pass HIV to others. However, they are nevertheless at risk of becoming infected through transfusion of contaminated blood or sexual mixing with people who practice high-risk behaviour. And young children are at risk of becoming infected from their mothers perinatally but are highly unlikely to spread HIV.

In a sexually-transmitted HIV epidemic, the speed at which HIV spreads from people with a large number of partners to those with very few partners depends on the extent of mixing between people with different levels of sexual activity. If people with large numbers of partners have intercourse only with others who are similarly active (known is assortative sexual mixing), then HIV will tend to rise rapidly within those groups but only very slowly and to a limited extent in the rest of the population.

As a result, the epidemic will achieve lower peak levels of infection in the entire population than if those with large numbers of partners also have sex with those who have fewer partners (known as random or disassortative mixing). Mixing patterns explain why HIV does not spread through a population at a uniform rate. Rather, it spreads in a series of smaller epidemics that race through overlapping subpopulations whose behaviour puts them at various degrees of risk, then outward to those with less-risky behaviour with whom they mix.

Sex workers whose clients do not use condoms, injecting drug users who share unsterilised injecting equipment and others with very high rates of partner change are typically the first to be infected in an HIV epidemic. HIV prevalence in these groups can rise very rapidly.

Some of the differences in the rate of increase across cities can be attributed to differences in the timing of the introduction of the virus. However, other factors also appear to be at work. HIV prevalence among sex workers in Santo Domingo, Dominican Republic, has risen more slowly; this is believed to be due to very high rates of condom use among brothel-based sex workers. HIV tends to move even more rapidly among injecting drug users who share injecting equipment than among sex workers because the risk of transmission per contact is much greater.

If there is very little mixing between people with different degrees of risky behaviour, the overall epidemic may have multiple peaks. Incidence may rise and fall several times as first one group and then another becomes nearly saturated by the virus. Thus, a sustained decline in incidence in a specific group of people with risky behaviour does not necessarily signal the end of the epidemic in the entire population.

Concurrent partnerships: Partnerships that overlap in time are concurrent partnerships. Examples of concurrent partnerships include: partnerships between married men or women and commercial or casual sexual partners; people engaging in long-term relationships with more than one casual partner; and polygyny, the practice of having more than one wife. In two populations in which individuals have the same average number of partners in a given period, HIV and other STDs will spread more rapidly in the population in which partnerships are concurrent than in the population in which partnerships occur sequentially.

This is because when partnerships are sequential, the virus cannot spread to a new susceptible person until the dissolution of one relationship and the start of another. In a concurrent partnership, it can infect more susceptible people in a shorter period of time.

The impact of heterogeneity, mixing and concurrency: The combined effect of heterogeneity in sexual behaviour, mixing between groups of different behaviours and concurrent partnerships can have a profound impact on the potential course of the HIV/AIDS epidemic. The four simulated populations are identical in every respect, except in their patterns of sexual behaviour, as follows:

— *Commercial and casual sex*: In this population, some men engage in commercial and casual sexual relationships before and after marriage; some women have relations with casual partners before marriage but all women are monogamous after marriage. The commercial and casual partnerships can be concurrent with each other and with marriage. Sex workers comprise about a one-fifth of 1 per cent of all women.

— *Commercial sex*: Some men engage in commercial sex before and after marriage with a small group of female sex workers comprising only one-quarter of 1 per cent of the female population. Neither men nor women have casual sexual relationships before or after marriage. Commercial and marital relationships can be concurrent.

— *Casual sex*: Some men and women have casual sexual relationships before and after marriage. There are no sex workers in this population, but casual partnerships can be concurrent with each other and with marriage.

— *Serial monogamy*: Some men have commercial and casual sexual relationships before marriage and some women have casual relationships before marriage. After marriage, neither men nor women have extramarital relationships. All relationships before marriage are serial; this is the only one of the four populations with no concurrent relationships. Sex workers are 0.05 per cent of the female population.

Most new cases of HIV infection at that point occur among people who have recently adopted high-risk behaviour. In the population in which there is casual but no commercial sex, the epidemic progresses more slowly, reaching a prevalence rate of only about 3 per cent eight years after the start of the epidemic. However, prevalence continues to climb, reaches 30 per cent and is still increasing 30 years after HIV is introduced. Finally, in the population that practices serial monogamy with commercial, casual and marital partners but no concurrent partnerships ("Serial monogamy," the lowest curve), HIV prevalence rises more quickly than in the population with only casual sex, but levels off at about 9 per cent. Thus, even without behaviour change to prevent HIV, the course of an HIV epidemic can be quite different across populations, depending on the heterogeneity of behaviour, the extent of mixing and the degree of concurrency in partnerships.

IMPLICATIONS FOR PUBLIC POLICY

The preceding description of how HIV/AIDS spreads through populations particularly the role that variations in individual behaviour play in determining the course of the epidemic, have important implications for government policies to prevent HIV.

Governments that invest in effective prevention before HIV/AIDS becomes evident can avert suffering, save lives and avoid potentially massive expenditures on AIDS treatment and care. There are several reasons why early intervention to change high-risk behaviour is preferable to later action. Early in an epidemic, HIV spreads exponentially. Because very few people are infected, the probability is greater that unprotected sex or needle sharing involving an infected person and a random partner will result in a new infection. Further, if the viral load is highest in the first months of infection, as scientists suspect, early in the epidemic a very large proportion of those infected will be, highly infectious.

Governments representing nearly half of the population of developing countries, 2.3 billion people-are in areas with nascent HIV/AIDS epidemics and are still in a position to act early and decisively to prevent a widespread epidemic. Among those countries are China, certain states of India, Indonesia, the Philippines, Eastern Europe, North Africa and the Middle East. Yet even in countries where HIV is already prevalent among those with risky behaviour, there are still opportunities for prompt intervention to prevent the spread of HIV into the next wave of people susceptible to infection.

Despite the compelling case for acting early, governments have often been slow to respond. This is understandable in those countries where HIV struck first, since very little was known in the 1970s and early 1980s about how HIV was transmitted and how its spread could have been prevented. In particular, the existence and implications of the long asymptomatic period of HIV infection were not well understood. Countries where the epidemic hit later have had the opportunity to benefit from increased knowledge about the disease and governments are becoming quicker to launch national AIDS prevention programs, no doubt due in part to the efforts of international programs like the Global Programme on AIDS and UNAIDS.

Yet even today, some policymakers dismiss the significance of a relatively small number of reported AIDS cases, not recognising that such a situation is precisely when prevention is needed. As recently as 1994, a senior health official in one populous developing country chided reporters that "to make a few thousand reported AIDS cases into an epidemic is just absurd." Tragically, such attitudes persist, despite the now widely understood fact that reported AIDS cases are but the tiny, visible portion of a deadly, mostly invisible and potentially explosive HIV epidemic.

There are many reasons why policymakers may be slow to confront HIV/AIDS. In virtually every country, the HIV/AIDS epidemic has been preceded by a period of denial. AIDS is perceived to be a problem of foreigners, an imported problem confined to tourists or to people who have lived abroad. Injecting drug use and unprotected sex with multiple partners are said to be problems only in other countries, not in one's own country.

The lack of reliable data on HIV prevalence and risk behaviour makes the potential for an epidemic easy to ignore. Even when officials and politicians understand that the conditions for an HIV epidemic exist in their country, they may be reluctant to raise the issue publicly or to initiate programs to prevent HIV among people engaged in high-risk behaviour, who are often stigmatised. Or, they may believe that the limited resources available would be better spent fighting more common health problems, such as tuberculosis and malaria.

Finally, officials and business leaders have sometimes attempted to conceal information about the extent of the epidemic because they fear it will discourage tourism or investment. Although some of these obstacles cannot be dismissed lightly, failure to overcome them and act early to prevent the spread of HIV can be extremely costly.

An HIV epidemic can only persist if the reproductive rate of HIV is greater than 1 in at least some subgroup of the population and if the shape of the epidemic is largely influenced by the degree of mixing between people with different degrees of risky behaviour. Other things being equal, those with the highest rates of partner change are most likely to contract and spread HIV. It follows that preventing HIV infection in someone with a high rate of partner change—sexual or injecting—will indirectly avert many more future infections than preventing infection in a person who practices low-risk behaviour and is thus less likely to infect others.

Therefore, for HIV, as for other sexually transmitted diseases, the most efficient strategy for reducing the spread of the disease is to prevent transmission among those with the highest rates of partner change. Prevention of infection among those with the highest rates of partner change has a "multiplier" effect in terms of preventing many more subsequent, secondary infections, most of them among individuals with low-risk behaviour.

The benefits of preventing transmission among those with the largest number of partners during the early stages of the epidemic have been well documented. However, as HIV spreads, an increasing number of new cases occur among people who are not themselves engaging in risky behaviour, but who nevertheless become infected by their partners. In fact, in advanced epidemics the majority of those infected may practice low-risk behaviour.

The long delay and higher prevalence rates notwithstanding, high condom use among those with the highest rate of partner change is still more effective in lowering prevalence in the whole population than is moderate condom use among men engaged in commercial and casual sex, who have fewer partners. Either of these strategies is far more effective than raising condom use among women in steady relationships. One can imagine other sexual behaviour regimes where condom use among sex workers might make less of an absolute difference than condom use in casual relationships, or where these levels of condom use in any one of the subpopulations or even in all of them combined are not sufficient to reverse the course of the epidemic.

Even so, interventions that prevent transmission among those with the highest rates of partner change will prevent more secondary cases per primary case averted than interventions that change only the behaviour of the population that practices low-risk behaviour It follows that, if interventions that reduce risky behaviour among those with the highest rates of partner change are not much more expensive per primary case averted than programs for low-risk populations, then they can be very cost-effective.

DISTRIBUTION OF HIV INFECTION IN DEVELOPING COUNTRIES

Developing countries find themselves at different stages of the HIV/AIDS epidemic due largely to differences in the timing of the introduction of HIV and in sexual and drug-injecting behaviour. Here we classify countries according to the level and distribution of HIV infection, which, as we shall see, has a significant influence on the cost-effectiveness of preventive interventions and on the scope of interventions to mitigate the impact of the epidemic. Despite the obvious value of a country typology, low-quality and inadequate data and our still-incomplete knowledge of the disease itself make any evaluation of a country's status very tentative.

Because collecting incidence data is very costly, HIV monitoring systems collect data on prevalence. However, prevalence data are rarely collected for representative samples of the population. Our typology is therefore necessarily based on prevalence among frequently monitored groups with presumed high-risk behaviour-sex workers, injecting drug users, homosexual and bisexual men, STD patients and the military risk-pregnant women attending antenatal clinics. Most of these groups present significant sampling problems.

Notwithstanding these and additional problems that we discuss below, by using available data from research studies and epidemiological surveillance, countries can be classified according to two broad criteria: first, the extent of HIV infection among groups of people often found to engage in high-risk behaviour and, second, whether the infection has spread to populations assumed to practice lower-risk behaviour. The typology includes three stages of the HIV/AIDS epidemic:

— *Nascent*: HIV prevalence is less than 5 per cent in all known subpopulations presumed to practice high-risk behaviour for which information is available.

— *Concentrated*: HIV prevalence has surpassed 5 per cent in one or more subpopulations presumed to practice high-risk behaviour, but prevalence among women attending urban antenatal clinics is still less than 5 per cent.

— *Generalised*: HIV has spread far beyond the original subpopulations with high-risk behaviour, which are now heavily infected. Prevalence among women attending urban antenatal clinics is 5 per cent or more.

Due to a lack of data, this typology does not address several important factors. In particular, it does not distinguish between countries based on incidence, the rate of new infections. As we have seen, because HIV cannot be cured and lasts many years, prevalence can rise even if incidence is declining. Prevalence data do not reveal whether the number of new infections is increasing, declining, or level, either in specific subpopulations or among the entire population. Moreover, prevalence data are available only for a few specific subpopulations.

Prevalence can stabilise in one or more of these subpopulations even as it spreads rapidly through others that are not monitored. These shortcomings highlight the importance to governments of collecting additional data on HIV incidence and prevalence so that policymakers can formulate an effective response. Even with much better data on incidence and prevalence, we would still lack sufficient behavioural information to confidently predict the course of the epidemic in a specific country.

Policymakers in most countries simply do not know how many people engage in commercial sex, casual sex, or injecting drug use; how frequently they do so; or the extent to which they take actions to reduce their risk of contracting HIV. Basic information on the levels of condom use and partner change among the general population is also unavailable. Without this information, it is simply not possible to accurately predict the course of the epidemic. For these reasons, we cannot predict with certainty in which low-prevalence countries HIV infection will take off or at what level prevalence will stabilise. Some countries where HIV is currently regarded as a minor problem may turn out to resemble eastern Africa, where the virus spread rapidly through groups with high-risk behaviour and widely into the general population. In other countries HIV may infiltrate groups with high-risk behaviour but never evolve into a generalised epidemic, even without intervention.

Knowledge of HIV may cause people to adopt less risky behaviour, with or without government urging. Countries with a high incidence and prevalence of STDs other than HIV are likely to be particularly vulnerable to a large and rapidly spreading HIV epidemic, because STDs and HIV are spread by the same behaviour and STDs enhance HIV transmission.

However, since most other STDs can be cured, countries with low STD prevalence may still have behaviour patterns that are conducive to the rapid spread of HIV. Lacking, the information to predict the course of the epidemic and given the terribly high human and financial costs of HIV/AIDS, it would be prudent to assume the worst and act aggressively to minimize the epidemic as early as possible. A list of countries and estimates of prevalence in different subpopulations are discussed below.

Africa

Ninety per cent of all HIV transmission in sub-Saharan Africa is by heterosexual sex. HIV has spread rapidly among people with high-risk behaviour and widely among those assumed to be at lower risk. Prevalence among urban sex workers exceeds 20 per cent in seventeen countries and is 50 per cent or more in nine countries. Infection rates among women attending antenatal clinics have grown rapidly to high levels in some areas, have stabilised at lower levels in others and appear to be declining in Kampala, Uganda. HIV has infected more than 5 per cent of women attending urban antenatal clinics in nineteen countries and in six countries more than 20 per cent are infected. An estimated two-thirds of all new cases of mother-to-child transmission worldwide occur in Sub-Saharan Africa.

The countries with generalised epidemics include most in eastern, southern and central Africa, plus Cote d'Ivoire, Benin, Burkina Faso and Guinea-Bissau in West Africa. There is often considerable geographic variation in infection levels within countries. Nigeria, which has more than 100 million people and is the region's most populous country, has areas at all three stages of the epidemic. In more than half of Nigeria's states the epidemic is concentrated. HIV has spread most widely in Lagos, along the west coast, Delta, Plateau, Borne and Jigawa states, located to the east and northeast.

However, in three states—Edo, Niger and Oyo—the epidemic is still nascent with low prevalence levels, even among subpopulations with high-risk behaviour. HIV was detected early in the Democratic Republic of the Congo (formerly Zaire), but in contrast to many eastern and southern African countries, prevalence has stabilised at less than 5 per cent on average in urban antenatal clinics. In

Uganda, one of the hardest-hit countries in Africa, HIV prevalence among young people has declined. Most Sub-Saharan African countries face the dual challenge of lowering HIV prevalence—which can happen only over many years—and of coping with the impact of existing high prevalence on the health system and society.

Domestic budgetary resources to accomplish this are quite limited. Countries with nascent epidemics in Sub-Saharan Africa—Cape Verde, Madagascar, Mauritania, Mauritius and Somalia—have a unique Opportunity to intervene early and aggressively to pre-empt a full-scale epidemic. High STD prevalence in Madagascar makes it vulnerable to the rapid spread of HIV. The epidemic in most of North Africa and the Middle East is also nascent, although there is evidence of rapidly climbing HIV infection among injecting drug users in Bahrain and Egypt, as has been the case in Asia.

Latin America and the Caribbean

More than half of the countries in Latin America and the Caribbean have concentrated epidemics. These include the most populous countries in the region—Brazil and Mexico. Six countries have nascent epidemics, two (Guyana and Haiti) have generalised epidemics and two (Bolivia and Panama) have insufficient information to be classified. Injecting drug use and sex between men have played a major role in transmission in many countries in Latin America. Roughly one-quarter of all HIV infections in Brazil (24 per cent, 1992) and a third in Argentina (39 per cent, 1991) have been attributed to transmission through injecting drug use, which is an important source of transmission in Uruguay as Well.

The epidemic is well established among homosexual and bisexual men in Argentina, Brazil, Colombia, Mexico and Peru and has infected significant numbers of sex workers in Argentina, Brazil, the Dominican Republic, Guyana, Honduras, Jamaica and Trinidad and Tobago. Although the data is limited, the relatively high prevalence of HIV among injecting drug users, homosexual and bisexual men and sex workers in Latin America suggests that in many of these countries the virus is poised to spread to the low-risk sexual partners of people who engage in high-risk behaviour.

In the Caribbean and parts of Central America, HIV is spread mostly through heterosexual transmission. Male and female cases are roughly equal in Haiti; the epidemic has spread broadly to 8 per cent of pregnant women and there is significant mother-to-child transmission. More than 70 per cent of AIDS cases in the Dominican Republic is attributed to heterosexual transmission; the ratio of male-to-female cases now stands at 2 to 1 and is declining.

HIV prevalence among pregnant women in that country has risen to a national average of 2.8 per cent and in some areas has reached 8 per cent. Following a similar path, 1 per cent of pregnant women in Honduras are also infected with HIV. In Guyana, which is in South America but faces on the Caribbean, nearly 7 per cent of women attending antenatal clinics were infected 1992.

Asia

In most Asian countries for which there is information, the epidemic has reached a concentrated stage either nationwide or at least in some states or provinces. This includes regions of the world's two most populous countries, China and India, most of Indochina and Malaysia. In the remaining Asian countries for which there is information, the epidemic is nascent; infection among those presumed to practice high-risk behaviour is less than 5 per cent.

Patterns of infection in east, south and southeast Asia have been greatly influenced by the proximity of many countries to the "Golden Triangle" of heroin production, located at the border between Laos, Burma and Thailand and to its distribution routes. HIV infection was first detected among those who inject drugs in Bangkok in 1987; during the next year it spread rapidly among injecting drug users in the Thai capital. The pattern was quickly repeated among injecting drug users in northern Thailand and along the border areas between southern Thailand and northern Malaysia. In 1989, HIV infection was identified in Myanmar Yunnan Province in China and in Manipur State in India.

HIV was detected among injecting drug users in Singapore in 1990.

Injecting drug use has been the main transmission mode in china where the most highly infected province, Yunnan, is adjacent to international drug routes. Male injecting drug users in Yunnan account for 78 per cent of HIV infections in China. In other Chinese provinces, infection rates are thought to be low, even among those who practice high-risk behaviour. Economic reforms that have helped to reduce the number of people in poverty in China by more than half since the late 1970s have also resulted in large increases in internal migration that could generate conditions conducive to the spread of HIV. Studies have estimated that nearly 100 million people, roughly one in twelve people in China, have moved either temporarily or permanently from their registered residence.

Much of the movement involves migration within provinces, but an estimated 20 million migrants have moved from poor areas of western China to eastern provinces. Most migrants are young, single, male, but many women have also migrated; some have reportedly come involved in prostitution. STDs, which were all but eliminated in China in the 1960s, are rising rapidly.

Early preventive interventions for migrants and sex workers in areas receiving migrants could reduce the likelihood of an epidemic of HIV and other STDs among these mobile groups. Among the nations of South Asia, the epidemic is believed to be spreading most rapidly in India and Pakistan.

In India, HIV is widespread among injecting drug users in the northeastern states of Manipur and Mizoram and is spreading to their sexual partners; prevalence in antenatal clinics in Manipur has reached 2 per cent. HIV is well established among sex workers and STD patients in much of southern India, including populous Maharashtra and Tamil Nadu states. In the city of Mumbai (formerly Bombay), HIV prevalence among pregnant women has reached 1 to 2 per cent.

In Pakistan, the infection rate among injecting drug users in Lahore was 12 per cent; as of 1995, HIV infection among women attending antenatal clinics was still extremely low. Transmission by those who inject drugs also may be a factor near a second major heroin-producing area, the "Golden Crescent," where Pakistan's Northwest Frontier meets the Badakhshan area of Afghanistan and the Baluchistan area of Iran. However, there are no recent data on HIV prevalence among drug users or other groups in these areas.

In Nepal, prevalence so far remains very low among injecting drug users in Katmandu. Bangladesh's HIV epidemic is still nascent, but, without behaviour change, HIV could spread quickly among a population of brothel-based sex workers and their clients. In most of southeast Asia, with the significant exceptions of Indonesia, Lao PDR, the Philippines and Papua New Guinea, the HIV epidemic is at the concentrated stage.

Injecting drug use has played a central role in the launching of HIV, often in conjunction with commercial sex, but heterosexual transmission is now the predominant mode of transmission. HIV is firmly established among injecting drug users and sex workers in Cambodia, Myanmar and Thailand and 1 to 3 per cent of pregnant women are HIV-positive in those countries. In Thailand, HIV prevalence peaked at 4 per cent among military conscripts in 1993, but has recently been declining following a national campaign to reduce sexual transmission of HIV through greater condom use and a reduction in commercial sex.

In Cambodia, however, infection levels in the military have reached nearly 7 per cent. In Malaysia and Vietnam, more than three-quarters of HIV infections are attributed to transmission through injecting drug use. Yet sexual transmission in Malaysia is clearly on the rise; nearly 40 per cent of HIV/AIDS cases seen at the University of Malaya Medical Center since 1986 were thought to be due to heterosexual transmission.

Rapid social change and economic dislocation that has accompanied the collapse of socialism in Eastern Europe and the former Soviet Union (FSU) have created a situation in which the potential for an HIV epidemic looms large. The available data on HIV prevalence suggest that most countries in the region are still in the nascent stage. However, reliable information on HIV prevalence by subpopulation is scarce in all but a handful of countries-almost two-thirds of all of the countries in this region cannot be classified based on the available information.

Ukraine has a concentrated HIV/AIDS epidemic, based on high HIV prevalence among injecting drug users; between January and August 1995, HIV prevalence among those who inject drugs rose to 13.0 per cent, from just 1.4 per cent. Just five months later, more than half of the injecting drug users in the Ukrainian city of Nikolayev were infected. A survey of new injecting users in Poland in 1995 found HIV prevalence of 4.7 per cent; a few years earlier, among longer-term injectors in the city of Warsaw the rate was 4.5 per cent. Given that those who inject drugs often travel to neighbouring countries, it is reasonable to expect a similarly rapid take-off among injecting drug users in the Russian Federation and Belarus.

In Romania, HIV initially spread primarily among children; over 90 per cent of AIDS cases in 1990 were among children under 13 years of age. It was erroneously believed that transfusing blood among children would provide important nutrients and boost the immune system. Instead, it spread HIV among them. The practice has since been abandoned. A key signal of the potential for an HIV epidemic in this region is the dramatic increase in STDs experienced by most countries since the collapse of the Soviet Union. The number of gonorrhoea cases has nearly doubled between 1990 and 1994 in four Eastern European countries. In Ukraine, the number of syphilis cases increased more than tenfold between 1991 and 1995.

Regardless of the stage of the epidemic, there are compelling reasons for governments to find ways to encourage people who practice risky behaviour to adopt safer practices as soon as possible. Fortunately, in most areas of the developing world it is not too late to avert a generalised epidemic. Half of the population of developing countries—2.3 billion people—live in areas where the HIV/AIDS epidemic is still nascent. Another third of the population of developing countries lives in areas where the epidemic is already concentrated but has yet to become generalised. In all these areas, action now to help people with the highest-risk behaviour protect themselves and others from HIV infection can save millions of lives and avoid massive future expenditures on AIDS treatment and care. Even in areas where the epidemic is already generalised, action to prevent infection among those most likely to contract and spread HIV can still make a substantial difference.

SELECTED READINGS

Antonucci, T. C. (1989), Social support influences on the disease process. In L. L. Carstensen & J. M. Neale (Eds.), *Mechanisms of psychological influence on physical health, with special attention to the elderly.* New York: Plenum Press.

Bandura, A. (1994), Perceived self-efficacy in the exercise of control over AIDS infection. In V. M. Mays, G. W. Albee, & S. F. Schneider (Eds.), *Primary Prevention of AIDS: Psychological Approaches.* Newbury Park, CA: Sage.

Barlett, J. G. (1993), *The Johns Hopkins Hospital guide to medical care of patients with HIV infection.* Baltimore, MD: Williams & Wilkins.

Broadhead, W. E., Kaplan, B. H., James, S. A., Wagner, E.H., Schoenbach, V. J., Grimson, R., Heyden, S., Tibblin, G., & Gehlbach (1983), "Reviews and commentary: The epidemiologic evidence for a relationship between social support and health". *American Journal of epidemiology.*

Burgess, A. P., Irving, G., & Riccio, M. (1993), "The reliability and validity of a symptom checklist for use in HIV infection: A preliminary analysis". *International Journal of STD & AIDS.*

Nicolosi, A., Leite, M. L., Musicco, M., Arici, C., Gavazzeni, G., & Lazzarin, A. (1994). "The efficiency of male-to-female and female-to-male sexual transmisstion of the human immunodificiency virus: A study of 730 stable couples". *Epidemiology.*

4

AIDS and Social Adjustments

It is a well documented fact that most people with HIV adjust after first learning they are HIV positive and continue adjusting over the course of infection. Coping is a process influenced by multiple competing stress factors including social discrimination, poverty and substance abuse, as well as an individual's social and coping resources. HIV-related coping is concerned with the thoughts and behaviours used in dealing with HIV infection. Coping constitutes cognitive and behavioural activities that serve to manage external and internal demands related to HIV infection that are seen as personally threatening. According to S.E. Taylor's cognitive Adaptational Model, adaptation to life-threatening illnesses is characterised by three general themes: a search for meaning, attempts to regain mastery or control over the illness and efforts to enhance self-esteem. Adjustment is a pervasive process and often involves distortions of reality in the service of psychological protection.

Models of cognitive behavioural coping also help explain adjustment to HIV infection. In general, these coping strategies comprise two broad clusters of coping behaviours: problem-focused coping and emotion-focused coping. Problem-focused coping includes cognitions and behaviours that actively seek resolution of specific stress factors (problem-solving coping). In contrast, emotion-focused coping is geared toward alleviating immediate distress and emotional turmoil without directly confronting sources of stress. In adjustment to chronic illness, coping falls within problem-focused and emotion-focused domains. Examples of illness-related problem-focused coping include seeking information about the disease, calling upon others for help and seeking medical advice and treatments.

Strategies for problem-focused coping are similar to confrontational coping behaviours and the "fighting spirit" observed among cancer patients. Emotion-focused coping is also common in serious medical illnesses, like HIV. Coping strategies must address a number of adaptational tasks in chronic illnesses, including harm reduction, tolerance of negative events, maintenance of positive self-image, establishing emotional equilibrium and maintenance of interpersonal relationships.

It is, however, important to note that illness-related experiences and coping processes differ for men and women and various ethnic groups and HIV risk populations. Adjustment to HIV infection can therefore be conceptualised as coping behaviours that occur within themes of searching for meaning, establishing a sense of control and enhancing self-esteem. Together, these themes and strategies provide a framework for understanding psychological adjustment to HIV infection.

Meaning, Control and Self-esteem

In her classic descriptions of cancer patients coping with their disease, S. E. Taylor described three themes in cognitive adaptation to chronic and life-threatening illnesses: meaning, control and restoring self-esteem. These dimensions also play important roles in adjustment to HIV infection.

Meaning is derived through an individual's efforts to understand adversity and human suffering. Perceptions of how one contracted HIV and beliefs about its implications can provide a sense of meaning. Searching for meaning may be conceptualised as an attempt to answer the question "Why me?". Causal attributions are one mechanism by which meaning is therefore ascribed.

Deriving meaning from a terminal illness like HIV is also influenced by many cultural and personal factors. A sense of meaning is not universally achieved by the terminally ill. When obtained, however, a sense of meaning can bring discovery of beneficial, self-affirming attitudes towards life in general and a new sense of self-knowledge or positive self- regard.

In a study of HIV-positive gay men, Schwartzberg found that HIV was perceived as a catalyst for personal growth. A greater appreciation for loved ones, reprioritising of values and time commitments and becoming more forgiving and less self-centered often occur after learning one is HIV-positive. Schaefer and Coleman also found that gay men with HIV infection gained a sense of meaning, purpose and value subsequent to testing HIV-positive. Relationships, self-discovery, aesthetic appreciation and contributing to the lives of others are all potential sources of meaning.

Control

Perceptions of control develop out of a sense of mastery that one has over one's illness. Uncertainties of chronic illness and diminishing perceptions of control are linked to psychological maladjustment. A sense of control buffers the effects of stressful life events and can lead to active coping to facilitate health and foster illness recovery.

A sense of control over stressful events emerges out of cognitions, coping strategies, attitudes and dispositions. Feelings of control over chronic illness can also develop out of a general personality style that leads to viewing events positively. Feelings of control over chronic illness seem necessary for psychological adjustment, even when perceptions of control are illusory.

Perceptions of control occur in multiple life domains, some of which are remotely affected by illness. Generally, a sense of control originates in one of two ways: internally or externally. Internal control, or personal control, stems from beliefs about actions that can change HIV disease progression. In contrast, external control involves beliefs that powerful external agents or forces control the course of HIV infection.

Internal control

A sense of personal control over stressful life events reduces psychological distress. Research has shown that perceptions of control over the course of disease correspond to psychological adjustment among people with HIV infection. The greater the uncertainty associated with a medical condition, the more important it is that people have a sense of control. Personal control over the course of illness is also associated with hope for longer survival and improved quality of life. S. E. Taylor et al. showed that perceived personal control plays a causal role in reducing psychological distress in chronic illness. A sense of control over the course of chronic illness can become maladaptive in some cases when such beliefs create a false sense of hope, particularly when efforts to control the disease are futile.

Still, most evidence suggests that feelings of control re-establish themselves despite the progression of a chronic illness. Perceived control persists even when situations become apparently uncontrollable. Personal control is durable because it joins with coping strategies. For example, perceived personal control and coping behaviours were associated in a study of almost 500 gay men in San Francisco. Using path analysis, Folkman et al. showed that perceptions of personal control correspond to a constellation of HIV-related coping strategies. A sense of control among HIV-positive men led to treatment involvement, including planed problem solving, advice and information seeking and positive appraisals. Similar findings were reported in a sample of 53 long-term AIDS survivors.

Although it can be seen as a belief or perception, personal control itself can take the form of a coping strategy. In this sense, a person may assume personal control over a particular aspect of illness. For example, compliance with medical treatments can be considered a form of control expressed as a coping strategy.

Control and coping can therefore appear similar to each other and often overlap. A sense of control and enacting problem-focused coping can also be related in the opposite manner, with coping strategies giving rise to a greater sense of personal control.

In an unusual example of how coping strategies can bring an increased sense of control, Schneider et al. found suicidal thoughts linked to AIDS-related events can function as a means of coping. It was *et al.* found that suicidal ideations may alleviate psychological distress, rather than emerging out of despair. Contemplating suicide helped some individuals continue functioning with a greater sense of personal control in relation to their future. This is not to suggest that all suicidal ideations occur to achieve a sense of personal control over HIV infection. Rather, this result illustrates that a need for control can be strong and may occur in subtle and unexpected ways.

The need to control one's own health decisions and physical functioning is observed when people first seek HIV antibody testing, as they enter early HIV infection and during later stages of AIDS. Control can be exerted over symptoms, HIV-related illnesses, the general course of HIV disease, or a combination of disease processes. S. E. Taylor et al. found that gay men in the Los Angeles MACS cohort sensed control over day-to-day symptoms, health maintenance and medical treatment. A sense of control over HIV-related symptoms corresponds to improved psychological adjustment particularly among those suffering moderate to severe symptoms.

Control may be exerted during HIV-related illnesses as well. Perceptions of control appear most adaptive when there is actual control available.

For example, individuals with HIV infection often engage in activities that have immediate and tangible health outcomes, including changes in diet, initiating an exercise program and seeking information about available treatments. One of the most common types of control exerted over the course of HIV involves taking responsibility for one's medical care. G. M. Reed et al. found that 79 per cent of gay men with HIV infection viewed themselves as having control over their medical care and control over the course of infection. Thus, a sense of control over illness progression has psychological benefits across phases of the HIV infection.

External control

External control beliefs involve forces outside the person thought to exert control over the course of illness. Individuals often believe that physicians and other medical professionals have a greater degree of control over the course of HIV than they do themselves. For example, one third of people with HIV infection believe that their physician has control over day-to-day symptoms and over two-thirds believe that physicians have some control over the course of infection.

Studies of non-HIV chronic illnesses show that perceptions of external control interact with illness-related factors to influence adjustment. In contrast, beliefs that others control the course of illness correlate with maladjustment among women with poor prognoses.

Control ascribed to powerful others is therefore related to adjustment only when others are credited with a positive outcome. Perceptions of medical professionals' control over HIV infection correspond with poor psychological adjustment, particularly when symptoms of HIV are advanced. People with HIV infection who believe others control their health and medical care are less well adjusted when compared with those who ascribe little control to external sources.

Medical care settings generally limit personal control, while facilitating the control of powerful others. Thus, perceptions of external control can be difficult to balance with perceived personal control when individuals are receiving medical treatment. Personal distress can especially occur when control is given over to physicians reluctant to take on HIV-related cases and who are perceived as lacking expertise in HIV disease. HIV infection has a poor prognosis and therefore understandably leads to distress when others are believed to be in control of one's fate.

Self-esteem

Changes in body image, physical limitations and loss of

social roles adversely affect the self-esteem of chronically ill patients. S. E. Taylor identified enhancing self-esteem as a theme in the adjustment to chronic and life-threatening illnesses. Self-enhancement is achieved by deriving personal benefit from illness experiences either by comparing oneself with others who are less fortunate or by focusing on aspects of the illness to make one feel well-off.

Taylor found that cancer patients tend to compare themselves with others who are doing worse rather than better than themselves to build up their self-esteem. Downward comparisons enhance personal perceptions by focusing on one's positive relative to other's negative experiences. Unfortunately, little research has been done to evaluate self-enhancement processes in HIV infection. Thus, although people with HIV infection appear to have similar issues of self-esteem as those observed among cancer patients, conclusions must be wit held until more research is available.

COPING STRATEGIES

Problem-focused and emotion-focused coping constitute different means to achieve psychological balance. The particular coping strategies that an individual with HIV infection may use is determined by multiple factors, including stage of illness, personal coping history and perceived available coping resources. For example, men living in urban gay communities have access to stable resources that facilitate coping with HIV infection. In contrast, people with HIV infection living in rural areas lack resources that facilitate adjustment. There is evidence that men and women, ethnic groups and HIV risk groups differ in their use of coping strategies. Unfortunately, not enough information is available to allow for conclusions about differences among patterns of coping across segments of the HIV epidemic.

Problem-focused coping

Problem-focused coping consists of behavioural and cognitive strategies aimed at solving problems and resolving conflicts and is used most in situations where a person has a sense of personal control; doing something is potentially constructive. Direct confrontation of symptoms is a common example of problem-focused coping in chronic illness.

Mobilisation against chronic disease has positive effects on psychological adjustment, global psychological well-being, self-esteem, emotional well-being, subjective health and certain aspects of physical functioning. People with HIV infection frequently engage in action-oriented coping behaviours and appear to find these strategies psychologically beneficial.

An active, "fighting spirit" style of coping relates to positive effects on HIV disease progression as well as to adjustment to HIV infection. However, these relationships are correctional and health outcomes are likely bi-directionally linked to problem-focused coping. That is, with improved health people feel better and have more energy to engage in activities that in turn promote a sense of positive well-being.

Examples of problem-focused coping include trying to learn more about HIV infection, seeking new treatments, focusing on healthy changes in life-style and making plans to access new therapies. An examination of responses to a coping scale completed by HIV-positive men and women showed that active, problem-focused coping strategies were frequently endorsed. Similarly, long-term survivors use a number of active coping strategies without any one dominant pattern of responses emerging. Broadly defined HIV-related active coping encompasses cognitive coping, involvement in medical treatment, seeking information, lifestyle changes and social activism.

Cognitive coping strategies

Problem-focused cognitive coping is characterised by attempts to achieve a perspective that protects against the graveness of HIV or creates meaning out of being HIV positive. People with HIV infection commonly adopt a life view that promotes a sense of emotional well-being. Typical cognitive techniques used by people with HIV include meditation, self-hypnosis and mental imagery. Plans of action and positive thoughts about the future are also common cognitive coping strategies. Fleishman and Fogel found that thoughts such as concentrating on how things could be worse and looking toward the brighter side of things were related to lower levels of depressive mood. Kalichman found that 62 per cent of HIV-positive men and women had rediscovered what was important in their lives after learning they were HIV positive and 67 per cent indicated that they rehearsed particular actions as a means of coping.

Table 1
Problem-focused coping strategies endorsed by people with HIV infection

Coping strategy	*(% endorsing item)*
Analysed the problem to understand it better	67
Talked with someone to find out more about the situation	62
Got professional help	45
Made a plan of action and followed it	49
Talked with someone who could do something concrete about the problem	51
Changed something so things would turn out all right	62
Came up with a couple of different solutions	55

Involvement in medical treatment

Becoming active in one's medical care can facilitate adjustment to HIV infection. Seeking medical treatments, becoming informed about possible treatment side effects, identifying opportunities to enroll in clinical trials and experimental treatments, exploring complementary therapies and developing alliances with medical professionals are examples of increased involvement. Participation in AIDS clinical trials offers additional psychological benefits, such as an increased sense of control and increased hope.

Information seeking

Identifying and consuming pertinent information are among the greatest needs expressed by the chronic medically ill and by people with HIV infection in particular. Namir, Wolcott, Fawzy and Alumbaugh found that 85 per cent of HIV-positive gay men had tried to find out more information about their illness. Information seeking is common in HIV infection, with over 62 per cent of HIV-positive men and women indicating that they have discussed with others ways to find out more about HIV and AIDS.

Sources of information vary and most people seek materials from multiple resources. Thus, a large number of information services have been established to meet these needs. Federal, state and local health departments, as well as activist and grass-roots organisations, have produced brochures, booklets and newsletters for people with HIV infection. Rapid changes in the development, testing and clinical trials of treatments for HIV infection and HIV-related opportunistic illnesses overwhelm people with information, particularly immediately after they test HIV positive.

Life-style changes

People with HIV infection often make changes in their life-style and everyday habits to promote their physical health. Namir et al. found that 81 per cent of HIV-positive patients began eating more healthily and taking vitamins in response to testing HIV positive. Individuals with HIV infection also report resting more and reducing their use of alcohol and drugs as a means of coping. Aerobic exercise is another common change in life-style that buffers stress for people with HIV infection. Changes in life-style bolster a sense of personal control in a similar fashion as do other problem-focused coping strategies.

Social activism

Although only 7 per cent of HIV-positive people become involved in political activism as a means of coping, those who are social activists experience benefits in terms of their psychological adjustment. Those who are not themselves activists may vicariously benefit from knowing others who are.

Action against HIV infection by way of problem-focused coping strategies occurs most frequently in response to the aspects of disease that appear controllable, such as medical care, health behaviour changes and social relationships.

The realities of HIV infection indicate that most benefits come from attempts to prevent opportunistic illnesses and control symptoms. Forestalling the onset of or curing opportunistic illnesses increases involvement in treatment, information seeking and life-style changes.

Emotion-focused coping

Emotion-focused coping consists of cognitive and behavioural adjustment strategies that do not directly intervene with problem situations. These coping strategies include denial, acceptance, avoidance, escape, distancing, use of distractions and positive reappraisal.

Chronic medical patients can benefit from certain emotion-focused coping strategies. One model of coping with terminal illness almost exclusively relies on emotion-focused coping. Kubler-Ross described five stages of adjustment to terminal illness and loss: denial, experience and expression of anger, bargaining with external forces perceived as controlling the course of illness, depression in the face of continued deterioration and acceptance.

Table 2

Emotion-focused coping strategies endorsed by people with HIV infection

Coping strategy	*% endorsing item*
Turned to work or substitute activity to take my mind off things	44
Looked for the silver lining; tried to look on the bright side of things	64
Told myself things that helped me to feel better	54
Didn't let it get to me; refused to think too much about it	45
Wished that I could change what happened or how I felt	54
Daydreamed or imagined a better time or place than the one I was in	61
Wished the situation would go away or somehow be over with	54
Reminded myself how much worse things could be	63

Given that emotion-focused coping is effective when a person can have little actual control over the course of illness, it is not surprising the Kubler-Ross's model revolves around emotion-focused coping. Consistent with Kubler-Ross's model, Kalichman found that people with HIV engage in denial, acceptance, avoidance and distractions as coping strategies. Table 2 presents the percentages of HIV-positive people in Kalichman's study who endorsed eight emotion-focused *coping* strategies.

Denial

Denial may occur at several points in HIV infection. For example, people may avoid getting tested for HIV antibodies despite high-risk histories or even illness symptoms. Following receipt of an HIV-positive test result, some people engage in denial by believing that HIV infection is not the cause of AIDS. Still others do not believe that their test results are accurate and may either get retested or just go on as if they were not tested in the first place. HIV infection may also be denied by misattributing symptoms to non-HIV-related causes. Although denial may recur over the course of HIV infection, few long-term survivors with AIDS use denial as a coping strategy. Leserman et al. found that denial among gay men with AIDS was associated with negative moods, particularly anger. Thus, denial can be an effective shelter against emotional distress, but precludes problem-focused coping.

Acceptance and resignation

Realistic acceptance was proclaimed by Kubler-Ross as a natural final stage of coping with terminal illness. Kubler-Ross described acceptance as a state of calm that is relatively void of negative and positive emotions. According to Kubler-Ross, however, acceptance does not necessarily represent a constant state, with a sense of acceptance fading in and out over the course of illness. Studies of patients with life-threatening illnesses show that acceptance and resignation are most common among those who have diseases with little chance of cure or long-term remission. These same descriptions seem valid in AIDS. Griffiths and Wilkins found that individuals diagnosed with HIV infection for five years or longer accepted their condition. Long asymptomatic periods of HIV infection may facilitate acceptance of impending illness. Over 54 per cent of people in one study had accepted being HIV positive and believed that nothing could be done to help them.

Accepting HIV infection is not, however, necessarily associated with psychological adjustment. G. M. Reed, Kemeny, Taylor, Wang and Visscher found that realistic acceptance of HIV infection was unrelated to a global index of psychological adjustment.

Reed *et al.* also found that individuals who were resigned to dying of AIDS demonstrated shorter lengths of survival. These findings suggest that personal acceptance of future debilitation, loss of functioning and death may be related to poorer psychological adjustment in HIV infection.

A possible reason for these findings is that acceptance and resignation are inconsistent with confrontational styles of coping and a fighting spirit, both of which are associated with problem-focused coping. Perhaps because AIDS represents multiple opportunistic illnesses, each of which may be successfully treated, AIDS patients believe and with good reason, that they can live longer if they just get past an AIDS-related condition.

Avoidance

For the most part, avoidance coping corresponds to psychological distress and poor long-term adjustment. Cognitive and behavioural avoidance occurs relatively frequently early in asymptomatic HIV infection as compared with later symptomatic phases. HIV symptomatics rarely use cognitive and behavioural avoidance strategies. Concern over health and existential issues correlate with use of avoidance coping. Like other medical conditions, avoidance coping in HIV infection leads to increased psychological distress and dysphoria. Avoidance coping includes simply trying to forget about being HIV positive, cancelling medical appointments and refusing to discuss HIV infection.

Distraction

Cognitive and behavioural distraction strategies seem to occur with greater frequency than avoidance techniques and, in contrast with avoidance, may facilitate psychological adjustment. In one study, 38% of HIV-positive people stated that they had gone on a vacation to cope and 44% turned to work or some other activity to distract themselves from thoughts of being HIV positive.

People with HIV infection report going out with friends, treating themselves to something special and thinking about things unrelated to their condition as means of distracting themselves from thinking about being HIV positive. Movies, theatre and music are also common means of distraction.

However, opportunities to divert attention away from being HIV positive diminish in advanced stages of HIV infection.

Substance use may provide a temporary escape from the everyday distress that can be associated with HIV infection, as well as an escape from symptoms and illness. Alcohol and drug use is common in gay communities and particularly frequent among men at risk for HIV infection. Unfortunately, little is known about baseline coping among individuals who later become HIV infected, particularly with reference to maladaptive coping. Wishful thinking and intellectualisation may also be used to feel better for the moment without directly addressing HIV infection.

OPTIMISM AND SPIRITUALITY

Beyond specific coping strategies, attitudes and personal styles are closely related to adjustment. A positive outlook toward the future and an importance placed on faith and spiritual beliefs may motivate coping responses. Optimism and spirituality are related to meaning, control and self-esteem. Optimism and hope parallel a sense of personal control and help foster a sense of self-esteem, whereas spirituality is more closely connected to a search for meaning.

Optimism and hope

For people facing adversity, positive beliefs about the future can promote a sense of self-worth and inner-strength. Optimism in relation to HIV disease corresponds to a greater sense of control and increased use of problem-focused coping. Knowledge of being HIV positive evokes a sense of optimism about not developing AIDS that is only seen in individuals who are HIV positive.

Perceived control over HIV infection can be characterised as unrealistically optimistic and serve psychologically self-protective functions. Like personal control, optimism gives rise to problem-focused coping and leads to improved adjustment.

Optimism and hope both consist of expectations that something positive lies ahead, imply confidence about the future and result in positive appraisals about potential illness outcomes.

In a study of HIV-positive gay and bisexual men, Pakenham *et al.* found that a sense of optimism was related to psychological adjustment. In addition to HIV-specific optimism and hope, a more global style of positive thinking, or dispositional optimism, may reduce fears and promote problem-focused coping. Dispositional optimism is associated with reductions in psychological distress, alleviation of worries and concerns about AIDS, decreased perceptions of risk of developing AIDS and the use of problem-focused coping. Long-term survivors with AIDS demonstrate a psychological resiliency that reflects dispositional optimism.

Rabkin, Remien, et al. found that long-term survivors were able to articulate goals and saw the future in a positive light. Thus, positive attitudes, optimistic outlooks and hope compose a constellation of attitudes that contribute to psychological adjustment in HIV, particularly among people at later stages of infection.

Spirituality

HIV-positive individuals possess a broad range of religious beliefs and diverse spiritual practices, including identification with long-held faith and inquiries into new spiritual expressions. Once again like other chronic illnesses, existential and spiritual issues emerge out of questioning how the personal tragedy of HIV infection could happen to anyone. Unlike other life-threatening illnesses, HIV infection is associated with behaviours opposed by many traditional religious institutions. People with HIV infection may encounter reprehension rather than support when seeking guidance from spiritual leaders. Thus, it is not uncommon for individuals with HIV infection to seek new and alternative modes of spiritual expression.

For example, Carson found that gay men with AIDS do not achieve spiritual well-being as a result of participating in formal religions, but rather through an individual's ability to respond to existential challenges. In another study of gay men with HIV infection, Somlai and Kalichman found that men who were ambivalent toward formal religious doctrines developed new and alternative modes of spiritual expression. Spiritual practices with immediate and tangible benefits were frequently reported in this sample of HIV-positive men and women.

Spiritual needs and practices are common among HIV-positive people, with more than half of participants in one study indicating that they frequently prayed, 40 per cent reporting they had found new faith and 62 per cent often hoping that a miracle would happen in relation to their being HIV positive.

Spiritual practices potentially provide multiple sources of comfort, including support from beliefs in connection with a higher power and social support from a spiritual community. Religiosity and spirituality can reduce the burdens of caregiving for partners of HIV-positive patients who are themselves HIV positive. Social support, whether through participation in spiritual practices or otherwise, constitutes an important dimension of adjustment in its own right.

On the basis of the literature and information gained from interviews with HIV-positive men and women the following ideas are offered to aid practitioners in promoting adaptive coping with HIV-positive clients.

People with HIV infection may be empowered to chart their own course of health care and medical treatment. Being HIV positive can lead to a sense of demoralisation and can halt most plans for the future. People with HIV infection may therefore require encouragement to exert control over their responses to HIV disease and become active participants in their medical treatment.

Asking questions and developing a treatment alliance with health care providers should be encouraged. Clinical trials and complementary therapies offer opportunities to become engaged in one's own treatment. Such actions may have positive effects on psychological adjustment as well as health status.

Coping can be facilitated by anticipating physical declines. It is important for people with HIV infection to recognise that coping and support needs change over the course of infection. Fatigue, weakness, illness symptoms and treatment side effects may interfere with psychological adjustment. A lack of initiative and physical disability interfere with coping at later phases of HIV infection. Recognising these changes before their onset affords the opportunity to build a safety-net of coping supports in advance of physical decline.

The availability and use of multiple coping strategies facilitates adjustment processes. Thus, individuals with a broader range of coping behaviours will have more coping options. Diversity and flexibility in coping allows ineffective coping responses to be replaced with new strategies, increasing the chances that coping will meet the needs of a given situation.

Distractions from HIV-AIDS decrease psychological distress. HIV infection can consume a person's entire being. Over the course of HIV disease, relationships are often lost and the ability to actively participate in life diminishes. HIV infection usually leads to physical limitations that result in unemployment and restricted social activities.

At the same time, regular medical visits increase, medications become routine and people are surrounded by others with HIV infection and AIDS. Opportunities for distractions become more constricted as the infection progresses. Social interactions and keeping busy become valued breaks from intrusive thoughts of being HIV positive. Clients with HIV infection appear to benefit from actions and practices that provide immediate and tangible coping outcomes. Recognising an ultimate end to one's life may create pressure to adjust. As the HIV epidemic progresses and more people die of AIDS, psychological numbing, complacency and hopelessness may replace a fighting spirit.

People with HIV infection should be encouraged to look toward future developments in treatment. Advances in antiretroviral and prophylactic treatments against opportunistic illnesses have increased survival periods for people with HIV infection. Although a cure for HIV infection that clears the virus from the body is not in sight, advances in preventing, treating and curing HIV-related illnesses are occurring at an astounding pace.

Denial is maladaptive when it interferes with medical treatment decisions and deters proactive health decisions. There are numerous ways that denial is used to cope with HIV infection. For example, some believe that HIV is not the cause of AIDS or that the HIV-antibody test has a high false-positive rate. Such beliefs inhibit seeking medical treatments that can extend and enhance the quality of life. Realistic optimism, as opposed to denial, can increase treatment seeking and promote proactive health decisions, as well as other problem-focused coping strategies.

Substance use as a means of avoidance is common, where alcohol and other drugs are used as an escape from daily life stress factors including HIV infection. Substance use can provide a temporary escape from emotional distress of HIV infection. Prolonged substance abuse, however, interferes with problem-focused coping, disrupts social relationships and work attendance and can become psychologically maladaptive.

Eliminating substance use as a means of coping requires adopting optional coping behaviours that meet immediate and tangible needs. Individuals who become substance dependant may require specialised treatment as well as a means of replacing substance use with adaptive coping behaviours. Interpersonal relationships can help to alleviate psychological distress associated with chronic and life-threatening illness. Social support promotes cognitive and behavioural coping, facilitates a sense of meaning, enhances self-esteem, fosters a sense of belonging and increases available coping resources.

Unfortunately, the chronically ill often lack adequate social support at a time when it is most needed. Depression and anxiety associated with chronic illness can further disrupt relationships and distance people from potential social support.

Social support is related to stress-health relationships, mortality and other health-related outcomes. Social support is defined here as a multidimensional construct that includes support needs, available resources and satisfaction. In addition, social support refers to multiple aspects of interpersonal relationships including the number and types of contacts a person has, the functional content of relationships and the perceived quality or adequacy of support. In relation to chronic illness, each dimension of social support tends to vary at different stages of disease. Two conceptual models of health-related social support are described in the literature: models that emphasise the main effects (or direct effects) of support and models that view social support as an immediate buffer of stress.

Main-effects models posit that social support directly increases health by information, enhanced self-esteem, or perceived control. Stress-buffering models, on the other hand, state that when a person is under duress, social support increases information, emotional well-being, or tangible resources that in turn affect health outcomes. Both models of support incorporate information, compassion and the assistance of others that are either directly or indirectly linked to health and illness.

Social support fosters a sense of purpose or meaning and promotes health behaviours, including treatment seeking and treatment compliance. Social support may also affect perceptions of stressful events and coping. Thus, there is considerable evidence that the structural and functional dimensions of support are important aspects of psychological adjustment to HIV-AIDS.

STRUCTURE OF SOCIAL SUPPORT

Social networks vary across the HIV epidemic. However, like most aspects of the epidemic, information about the structure of social support has come from studies of primarily cancasian, middle-class, gay and bisexual men. This bias in the literature may be particularly troublesome because social networks of gay men are qualitatively different from those of heterosexuals and gay communities have in many places organised to support people with AIDS.

Greater support is received by men more closely identified with gay communities, as opposed to bisexual men and men outside of gay social networks. Although social networks within gay communities differ from those of other population segments, the benefits of social support do not differ. Gay communities themselves are heterogeneous, with differences, for example, in social support among ethnic groups. Ostrow et al. found that African American gay men benefit less from social support and report less affirming social networks than their white counterparts. These differences may exist because social support networks vary in terms of ethnic composition and social classes. For example, African Americans as a group exhibit social support structures that reflect cultural differences in help-seeking behaviours and informal support. Factors related to accessing community resources influence ethnic and cultural differences in social support. Similarly, Latin Americans and other ethnic minorities exhibit diverse patterns of social networks and the social networks of women differ from those of men. Injection drug users often lack support in their relationships. Opportunities for social support are reduced by unemployment, poverty, isolation and other factors related to social disadvantage. Social stigmas, loss of financial resources, changes in self-image and alienation from peer groups are all aspects of HIV infection that affect the availability of and satisfaction with social support.

Depression and psychological distress, fear that others will discover one's condition and concerns of transmitting the virus promote isolation. Even before learning they are HIV positive, however, many HIV-positive people compartmentalise their social networks.

Relationship partners

Relationship partners are a primary source of social

support. As in other chronic medical conditions, support from a spouse or long-term relationship partner is an important aspect of effective social support systems in HIV infection. Unfortunately, support offered by relationship partners is often threatened by HIV infection. In particular, sexual relations and pair bonding can deteriorate when one or both partners are HIV positive. Sexual relationships can become strained because of declines in health, as well as fears of transmitting HIV. Independent of caregiving, additional burdens are placed on partners who are themselves HIV positive.

Friends and peers

Social support networks in HIV infection consist primarily of friendships and peer relationships. Friends are the main source of social support among gay and bisexual men and among injection drug users. Friends offer empathy, accessibility and shared values and culture and friendships are associated with psychological adjustment among people with HIV infection. Integration into a community that is sensitive to the needs of those with HIV infection increases the number of HIV-positive peers one has.

As the HIV epidemic expands, numerous community-based organisations have emerged to bring people with HIV infection together. Relationships among people with HIV are grounded in common experiences that break down barriers of ignorance and stigmatisation.

Family support

Family relationships typically provide stable support during chronic illness despite the disruptions caused to family continuity. Stigmas that predate HIV infection create unfortunate barriers to family support. For example, Donlou et al. found that gay men with HIV infection did not perceive their families as helpful in their efforts to cope with being HIV positive. Family estrangement can be closely related to a long history of rejection.

Families are being called on to assume greater responsibilities for caregiving, particularly at the later phases of infection. Caring for an ill person is a highly stressful role. Chronic illness has similar psychological affects on family caregivers as on patients themselves. Family caregivers report high levels of distress, with over 75 per cent of parent caregivers experiencing symptoms of depression and 74 per cent of siblings having repeated thoughts of death and dying. Parents experience distress from the uncertainties of HIV disease and from witnessing its deteriorating effects over a long period of time. Parental caregiver stress is obviously compounded when the parent himself or herself is HIV positive and he or she is caring for their HIV-infected child.

Professional caregivers

Significant demands are placed on professional caregivers of people with chronic illnesses. In addition to the usual stress of working with terminally ill patients, HIV infection involves social stigmas, prejudices and biases. Like other chronically ill patients, people with HIV often express anger toward professional caregivers. Professional caregivers are crucial to social support systems in HIV infection. Although relationship partners, friends and family provide emotional support and assistance with daily tasks, professional helpers are perceived by people with HIV as a critical link to health-related information resources and advice. Access to information is an important feature of professional caregiver relationships.

Disclosure, reciprocity and loss

Social support can be available without disclosing HIV status, but to receive support related to HIV infection, individuals must disclose. Difficulties associated with HIV-status self-disclosure include fears of rejection and social isolation that can occur at times when needs for social support are greatest. Difficulty disclosing HIV status is common, even to sexual partners, where there is a moral obligation to do so.

Opportunities to reciprocate support are another important dimension to feeling supported. Providing social support can buffer stress to an even greater extent than receiving support. For example, reciprocity decreases hostility and depression among some people with HIV infection. Various sources of loss associated with HIV infection, including unemployment, rejection and deaths of friends, attenuate social support by shrinking the size of social networks. Illness and death of relationship partners, friends and acquaintances constrict social contacts and therefore reduce opportunities to gain and reciprocate support. Among population subgroups hit hardest by AIDS, relationship losses have been devastating. Paradoxically, by becoming connected to a supportive network, such as through an service organisation, an activist group, or a support group, a person increases their risk of losing relationships and constricting support that they have come to rely on.

Relationships with committed partners, friends, peers, family members and professional helpers form a structure and context of social support. Ethnic, cultural and gender differences in social networks and social stigmas in HIV infection, create barriers to support, increasing isolation among people who most need support.

To gain support and opportunities to reciprocate, HIV-positive individuals must overcome barriers and selectively self-disclose. Although numbers and frequencies of social contacts are related to the availability of support, the content of relationships and the actions of others determine the support that a person receives.

FUNCTIONAL DIMENSION OF SOCIAL SUPPORT

Feeling supported is determined by more than mere social contact. Social interactions must address the demands of stressors if they are going to protect against emotional distress. Theories of social support traditionally encompass three functions that buffer stress and promote psychological well-being: emotional, informational and instrumental support. Emotional support consists of affection, comforting and encouragement that result in positive effects on self-esteem feelings of self-worth and a sense of belonging. Informational support, such as advice or updated knowledge, may help people interpret, comprehend, or cope with HIV infection. Finally, materials, assistance and services have practical functions and constitute an instrumental dimension of support.

Relationships can establish and maintain emotional balance and are therefore considered a high priority in coping with HIV. Emotional support, like emotion-focused coping, does not directly address matters that affect HIV progression or the symptoms of HIV infection. Emotional support does, however, enhance psychological well-being by building hope and optimism. One emotional support need identified by people with HIV infection is physical contact. Touch communicates not being afraid of casual HIV transmission and can be a symbol of acceptance and understanding. Having a confidant is another type of emotional support that promotes well-being.

Uncertainties of HIV infection can cause a strong need for information. Accurate information can lead to realistic expectations about the course of illness, which may in turn facilitate psychological adjustment. People with HIV infection may seek information about their prognosis, health care and treatment options, insurance coverage and so forth. Gathering information contributes to a sense of control and contributes to problem-focused coping.

Instrumental support

Practical assistance with everyday needs helps to reduce distress and increase positive health appraisals. In some circumstances, instrumental support can have greater psychological benefits in HIV infection than either emotional or informational support. The availability of assistance can relieve stress caused by physical limitations. As has been the case with other psychological dimensions of HIV infection, the need for and availability of instrumental support, as well as other types of social support, changes over the course of HIV infection.

Social Support over the Course of HIV Infection

After initially testing HIV positive, individuals tend to be in crisis and benefit most from strong emotional and informational supports, which are unfortunately often unavailable because of fears, stigmas and attitudes toward sickness, death and AIDS. Initial responses from post-HIV antibody test counsellors and AIDS service organisations usually offer assistance when there are few other sources.

After the initial receipt of test results and as HIV infection progresses, the need for multiple types of support from multiple sources increases.

Fatigue, diminished self-esteem, physical disability and illness reduce an individual's ability to maintain interpersonal relationships. Illness therefore brings dissatisfaction with support even when it is available. Hays et al. found that satisfaction with informational support affected psychological adjustment but depended on the number of HIV symptoms a person had.

Gay men with more symptoms and less informational support were most depressed in relation to men with few symptoms and high informational support. Thus, informational support appeared to buffer the stress associated with developing symptoms. Relationships between social support and illness suggest that individuals who are most in need of support are therefore inclined to be dissatisfied with the support that they receive. Decreased availability of social support at later phases of HIV infection contributes to anger, resentment, hopelessness and depression. HIV infection invariably leads to hospitalisations, disabilities, unemployment and fatigue, all of which contribute to social isolation.

People in one's support networks may die from AIDS, others become emotionally exhausted and still others turn away from sickness and anticipatory loss. People with AIDS therefore seek support from multiple sources, particularly when compared with their asymptomatic HIV-positive and HIV-negative counterparts (Hays). Attempting to meet increased needs for support, AIDS service organisations, mental health and medical providers and others have derived a host of social support interventions modelled after programs for other chronic and life-threatening illnesses.

SOCIAL SUPPORT INTERVENTIONS

Interventions for individuals affected by the HIV epidemic provide emotional, informational and instrumental support. The most organised and accessible interventions have thus far included support groups, volunteer programs and hospice services.

Support groups

Support groups for people with HIV infection and their caregivers are similar to those for other medical patients. Groups have been used to foster interpersonal relationships that benefit people with HIV infection and those who provide their care. To date, there has been only one published clinical trial that tested different models of support for HIV-positive therapy clients. Kelly, Murphy, Bahr, Kalichman, et al. randomly assigned 68 HIV-positive (non-AIDS) men with heightened depressed moods to one of three experimental treatment conditions: a cognitive-behavioural treatment group, a social support group and an individual psychotherapy comparison condition and described the cognitive- behavioural condition as follows:

> The cognitive-behavioural groups focused on the use of cognitive and behaviour strategies to reduce maladaptive anxiety and depression. Each session had a behavioural or skill training theme and the sessions involved teaching participants the skill, group discussion of potential uses and benefits of the skill and weekly review of success in implementation. Skill areas included modification of cognitions that exacerbate anxiety or depression, progressive muscle relaxation, imaginal and cue-controlled relaxation, disclosure of serostatus and safer sex practices if sexually active and establishment of a network of socially supportive relationships. Participant questions, concerns and problems in implementation of change were handled from a cognitive problem-solving perspective. Most sessions also included at-home practice assignments.

In describing the social support group condition, they also stated that, the support group condition was modelled after the type of social support groups commonly used in coping with other types of illness (such as cancer) and often offered to HIV-positive persons by community AIDS service programs. Leaders of the support groups encouraged members to describe their feelings about having HIV infection; to identify shared problems, concerns, fears and hopes; to discuss how these issues are handled; and to adopt supportive and encouraging roles toward others in the group. There was considerable member-initiated discussion of how problems related to HIV were handled and participants were encouraged to share with and learn from, experiences raised by others in the group.

The group members generated the discussion topics of each session. Members often chose to talk generally about how it felt to have the group as a place to share with others their concerns about HIV. Skills training, behaviour rehearsal, contracting and practice assignments were not employed in this condition.

Results of the study showed that both support group models positively affected group members relative to the control group. However, the social support group appeared to have the greatest benefit over a 3-month follow-up period. Eighty-six percent of the social support group participants demonstrated clinically significant improvement on an index of distress severity, whereas two thirds of the comparison condition showed clinical deterioration, regressing below baseline levels during 3 months. Although members of the cognitive-behavioural group demonstrated a pattern of clinical change that was intermediate between the social support group and the control condition, cognitive-behavioural group participants did decrease their use of illicit substances to a greater degree than the other two groups.

The social support group allowed more time for emotional support and therefore emotion-focused coping, the cognitive-behavioural group emphasized problem-focused and active coping skills training. Thus, emotional adjustment was greatest among the social support group members, whereas declines in maladaptive coping behaviours occurred among the skills training participants.

Emotional support

Support groups can help people with HIV infection achieve a sense of emotional balance. Emotion-focused support groups emphasize hope, opportunities to gain insights from others, emotional catharsis and interpersonal connectedness. Mathews and Bowes identified several dimensions of effective HIV-related support groups, including sharing common experiences, group cohesiveness, reinforcing hope, helping others and learning from others' experiences.

Support groups also provide opportunities to deal with immediate crises. Psychosocial problem solving often occurs naturally in support groups.

Informational support

Support groups can include information dissemination pertinent to HIV infection and treatment. Alternatively, groups can focus exclusively on delivering and exchanging information, providing a forum for people with HIV infection to share experiences, knowledge and ideas. Knowledgeable group facilitators can become a primary source of information. There are several examples of information-based support groups.

Coleman and Harris conducted a psycho-educational support group to meet five specific information needs: information pertaining to HIV disease; management of health problems; health care and health insurance concerns; nutrition and its role in HIV infection; and issues of sexuality and intimate relationships.

Similarly, Hedge and Glover described an informational support group that focused on general health, stress, diet, medications, the medical system, legal issues, relationships, safer sex, complementary therapies and life-style changes brought about by HIV infection.

The information content of sessions and the information needs of group members vary during the course of HIV infection. In the context of a support group, people receive information along with emotional support, as well as have the chance to share information with others, therefore reciprocating support.

Structure and format of support groups

An important issue is group composition. Mixing clients who recently tested HIV positive with those who have been HIV positive for a long time, versus limiting groups to individuals at a particular phase of HIV infection, affects the issues addressed by the group.

Certain types of support are needed after initial diagnosis compared with during symptomatic illness. Including recently diagnosed people and long-term survivors in the same group allows the newly diagnosed to gain emotional and informational support from those who have "been there" and survived HIV infection. On the other hand, the newly diagnosed can become distressed when confronted by AIDS. Decisions regarding group composition therefore shape many of the issues that arise in sessions.

Other decisions include whether to mix groups or keep them homogeneous with respect to gender, sexual orientation and modes of having contracted HIV infection. Although homogenous groups are often considered more effective, there are benefits to diversity.

Professional versus peer facilitators, co-facilitators versus a single facilitator, whether to invite outside speakers and the degree to which group members and facilitators should be matched for sexes, ethnicity and HIV status are issues that require careful consideration. Unfortunately, there have been few empirical studies to guide these decisions. One study reported interviews that focused on the experiences and perceptions of support groups for people with HIV infection. All of the interview participants who had known they were HIV positive for more than a few months had attended at least one support group offered by AIDS service organisations. It was almost universal that the emotional tone of support groups influenced participant satisfaction. Most desired groups focused on positive attitudes and hope, rather than expression of negative feelings and sharing the perils of HIV infection. Information exchange was another critical factor in the perceived effectiveness of support groups. Information, including that shared by fellow support group members, was considered among the greatest benefits. Emotional support is gained from the feeling of not being alone. Groups can foster friendships and opportunities for activities or social events.

With respect to group composition, Kalichman found that the majority of gay men and heterosexual women felt comfortable coming to a mixed group and believed that diversity facilitated support. However, heterosexual men and injection drug users felt that their issues were different from those of gay men and heterosexual women and preferred separate groups.

Perceptions of mixing different phases of HIV infection depended on stage of illness. Those early in the course of HIV infection felt that they could benefit from the experience of people who had been HIV positive longer. For example, one man who had been HIV positive for 5 years stated, "There is a lot of support in seeing someone who has survived a long time with HIV and hear their stories." On the other hand, those at later phases believed that the newly diagnosed could offer emotional support and encouragement, but to a lesser degree than other long-term survivors.

Support groups for caregivers and the bereaved

Groups can meet the support needs of caregivers and people bereaved from AIDS. Caregiver support groups afford the opportunity to reflect, express and reconcile feelings related to caring for the ill. Support groups for caregivers are therefore geared toward sustaining emotional well-being to enable caregivers to continue their care. Like groups for people with HIV infection, caregiver support groups require addressing multiple losses. Helping people with HIV infection means repeated exposure to death and dying. Goals for professional caregiver support groups may include stress reduction to prevent burnout, reinforcing values that promote continued work with HIV-positive clients, enhancing and maintaining compassionate care and establishing professional boundaries with clients while fulfilling caregiver responsibilities.

The death of a person to AIDS results in bereavement similar to that found in loss from other chronic illnesses. Support groups assist survivors in rebuilding their lives.

The need for support during bereavement is well recognised. Lennon *et al.* found that grief reactions were greatest among those who had cared for a friend dying of AIDS who did not have their own support system.

In addition, 31 per cent of the men in the Lennon *et al.* study indicated that they did not receive adequate instrumental support when providing care for their friend and were not receiving emotional support while grieving. There have been few systematic studies of support groups for individuals who have suffered AIDS-related losses. In one small study, three men and four women who suffered a personal loss because of AIDS participated in a support group based on cognitive and behavioural coping strategies.

A nine-session support group focused on identifying and expressing emotions, developing adaptive coping strategies, increasing feelings of support, reducing psychological distress and avoiding maladaptive coping behaviours. Sikkema et al. found that the support group significantly reduced depression, grief reactions, anxiety, somatisation and other signs of distress.

The group participants benefited from focusing on specific rather than global stressors, support offered by fellow group members and their own emotional expression. Although it was based on a small sample without a control group, the study showed evidence for the potential value of support groups for those who suffer an AIDS-related loss.

Volunteer programs

AIDS service organisations that provide support to people with HIV infection rely on volunteers, many of whom are HIV-positive themselves. For example, programs may designate a buddy to provide one-to-one support for a person with HIV infection. Buddy volunteer programs provide both companionship and physical assistance. Volunteers visit and telephone others with HIV infection as well as provide instrumental support by shopping, cleaning, cooking and transportation.

When individuals with HIV infection themselves volunteer to help others, they have the opportunity to gain support from a network of fellow volunteers as well as the reciprocity of support offered by these relationships. Volunteer experiences can increase self-esteem, enhance personal worth and give a sense of meaning.

Terminal care and hospice

Hospice is an interdisciplinary approach to caring for patients with terminal illnesses, where recovery is unlikely and a prognosis is stated in months or weeks. Hospice care emphasizes the quality rather than quantity of life, holistic approaches to pain control that include psychological and spiritual pain and the involvement of family and others in the care of the patient. Hospice care also supports caregivers; by providing respite and convalescent care.

Another important aspect of hospice is its emphasis on palliative care. Palliation is a specialised form of care for patients with advanced progressive diseases where curative treatments are no longer feasible. Thus, hospice care integrates psychological, social and medical approaches to address the multidimensional issues of the terminally ill.

The progressive and terminal nature of HIV infection places it within the scope of the hospice mission. Unfortunately, many traditional hospices have been unwilling to accept AIDS patients into their services. The reluctance to care for people with AIDS has primarily been because of conflicts between aspects of HIV disease and eligibility criteria for hospice care. For example, people with AIDS often do not have a family member or friend willing to be designated as a primary caregiver, a necessity for hospice home care.

Moreover, AIDS has a largely unpredictable course, with sudden changes and reversals of life-threatening conditions. Additional problems may occur in relation to characteristics of certain AIDS patients, such as the continued use of illicit drugs. These aspects of AIDS set the disease apart from other chronic illnesses serviced by most hospice agencies. Thus, hospices have been started to exclusively care for people with AIDS. In general, the same hospice care is delivered, including an emphasis on pain control and quality of life, while offering specialised care for AIDS.

Interpersonal relationships can help to alleviate psychological distress associated with chronic and life-threatening illness. Social support promotes cognitive and behavioural coping, facilitates a sense of meaning, enhances self-esteem, fosters a sense of belonging and increases available coping resources. Unfortunately, the chronically ill often lack adequate social support at a time when it is most needed. Depression and anxiety associated with chronic illness can further disrupt relationships and distance people from potential social support.

Social support is related to stress-health relationships, mortality and other health-related outcomes. Although some studies have suggested that social support impedes disease progression, most research has focused on the role of social support in emotional adjustment. As a construct, social support lacks generally accepted operational definitions. Social support is defined here as a multidimensional construct that includes support needs, available resources and satisfaction. In addition, social support refers to multiple aspects of interpersonal relationships, including the number and types of contacts a person has, the functional content of relationships and the perceived quality or adequacy of support. In relation to chronic illness, each dimension of social support tends to vary at different stages of disease. Under this conceptualisation, perceptions of adequate social support will, by definition, enhance a sense of feeling cared for, loved, informed and affiliated.

Two conceptual models of health-related social support are described in the literature: models that emphasize the main effects (or direct effects) of support and models that view social support as an immediate buffer of stress. Main-effects models posit that social support directly increases health by information, enhanced self-esteem, or perceived control.

Stress-buffering models, on the other hand, state that when a person is under duress, social support increases information, emotional well-being, or tangible resources that in turn affect health outcomes. Both models of support incorporate information, compassion and the assistance of others that are either directly or indirectly linked to health and illness. Structural aspects of support include the frequency of social contacts, the relationships that serve as sources of support, the opportunity to reciprocate support and the integration of the individual into a supportive network. Individual differences in perceived social support, personality dispositions and the match between support and needs interact to determine the ultimate effects of social support. Figure 1 summarises the structural and functional components of social support. Independent of or in conjunction with coping strategies, these factors play an important role in psychological adjustment to HIV infection.

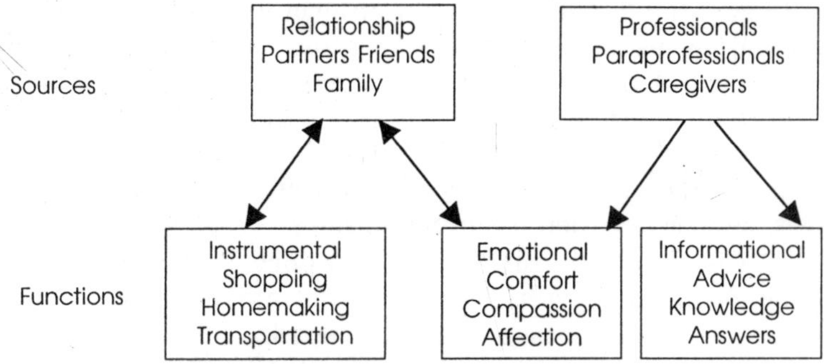

Fig 1: The structural and functional components of social support

Structurally, having a spouse or domestic partner, the frequency of social contacts, formal and informal group memberships and the number of close friends influence adjustment. Functionally, the content of social relationships affects health. Social support fosters a sense of purpose or meaning and promotes health behaviours, including treatment seeking and treatment compliance. Social support may also affect perceptions of stressful events and coping. Thus, there is considerable evidence that the structural and functional dimensions of support are important aspects of psychological adjustment to HIV-AIDS.

Like most aspects of the epidemic, information about the structure of social support has come from studies of primarily white, middle-class, gay and bisexual men. This bias in the literature may be particularly troublesome because social networks of gay men are qualitatively different from those of heterosexuals and gay communities have organised to support people with AIDS.

Although social networks within gay communities differ from those of other population segments, the benefits of social support do not differ. Gay communities themselves are heterogeneous, with differences, for example, in social support among ethnic groups. These differences may exist because social support networks vary in terms of ethnic composition and social classes.

For example, African Americans as a group exhibit social support structures that reflect cultural differences in help-seeking behaviours and informal support. Factors related to accessing community resources influence ethnic and cultural differences in social support. Similarly, Latin Americans and other ethnic minorities exhibit diverse patterns of social networks and the social networks of women differ from those of men. Injection drug users often lack support in their relationships.

Opportunities for social support are reduced by unemployment, poverty, isolation and other factors related to social disadvantage. Social stigmas, loss of financial resources, changes in self-image and alienation from peer groups are all aspects of HIV infection that affect the availability of and satisfaction with social support.

Depression and psychological distress, fear that others will discover one's condition and concerns of transmitting the virus promote isolation. Even before learning they are HIV positive, however, many HIV-positive people compartmentalise their social networks. For example, gay men commonly have two sets of friends, gay and heterosexual and two sets of family members, those who do and do not know their sexual orientation.

Similar partitioned relationships also occur among injection drug users and low-income women. Although segmentation may lead to reduced social contacts, the actual number of contacts per se is less important in psychological adjustment than is the quality of contacts. The most common sources of social support to people with HIV-AIDS include four types of caregivers: relationship partners, friends, family and professional caregivers.

Relationship partners are a primary source of social support. As in other chronic medical conditions, support from a spouse or long-term relationship partner is an important aspect of effective social support systems in HIV infection. Unfortunately, support offered by relationship partners is often threatened by HIV infection. In particular, sexual relations and pair bonding can deteriorate when one or both partners are HIV positive. For example, Agle, Gluck and Pierce found that hemophiliacs suffer sexual relationship problems, with over half of those studied feeling concerned about potentially transmitting the virus to their partners.

Similar issues arise for other subgroups of HIV-positive people. Sexual relationships can become strained because of declines in health, as well as fears of transmitting HIV. Independent of caregiving, additional burdens are placed on partners who are themselves HIV positive. Depressed mood and life disruptions occur among HIV-positive gay men who provide care to their partner. The stress of HIV infection can cause an end to long-term relationships.

Social support networks in HIV infection consist primarily of friendships and peer relationships. Friends are the main source of social support among gay and bisexual men and among injection drug users. Friends offer empathy, accessibility and shared values and culture and friendships are associated with psychological adjustment among people with HIV infection. Integration into a community that is sensitive to the needs of those with HIV infection increases the number of HIV-positive peers one has. As the HIV epidemic expands, numerous community-based organisations have emerged to bring people with HIV infection together. Relationships among people with HIV are grounded in common experiences that break down barriers of ignorance and stigmatisation.

Family relationships typically provide stable support during chronic illness despite the disruptions caused to family continuity. Stigmas that predate HIV infection create unfortunate barriers to family support. Family estrangement can be closely related to a long history of rejection. Hays, Chauncey et al. found that HIV-negative as well as HIV-positive gay men perceived their parents and siblings as the least supportive people in their lives. However, Hays et al. also reported that 92 per cent of gay men with AIDS sought help from family members, a higher number than both asymptomatic HIV-positive and HIV-negative gay men. Families are being called on to assume greater responsibilities for caregiving, particularly at the later phases of infection.

Caring for an ill person is a highly stressful role. Chronic illness has similar psychological affects on family caregivers as on patients themselves. Family caregivers report high levels of distress, with over 75 per cent of parent caregivers experiencing symptoms of depression and 74 per cent of siblings having repeated thoughts of death and dying. Parents of HIV-positive gay men and hemophiliacs worry about their child's health. Parents experience distress from the uncertainties of HIV disease and from witnessing its deteriorating effects over a long period of time.

Parental caregiver stress is obviously compounded when the parent himself or herself is HIV positive and he or she is caring for their HIV-infected child. Dual patient and caregiver roles are problematic in HIV infection because HIV-positive parents tend to be socially isolated. Thus, family support can contribute to the adjustment of individuals with HIV infection, but caregiving involves considerable emotional costs to families.

Significant demands are placed on professional caregivers of people with chronic illnesses. In addition to the usual stress of working with terminally ill patients, HIV infection involves social stigmas, prejudices and biases. Like other chronically ill patients, people with HIV often express anger toward professional caregivers. Para-professionals and volunteers who offer support experience similar types of reactions.

Thus, caregivers of HIV-infected loved ones require support themselves. Professional caregivers are crucial to social support systems in HIV infection. Although relationship partners, friends and family provide emotional support and assistance with daily tasks, professional helpers are perceived by people with HIV as a critical link to health-related information resources and advice. Access to information is an important feature of professional caregiver relationships.

Social support can be available without disclosing HIV status, but to receive support related to HIV infection, individuals must disclose. Difficulties associated with HIV-status self-disclosure include fears of rejection and social isolation that can occur at times when needs for social support are greatest. Difficulty disclosing HIV status is common, even to sexual partners, where there is a moral obligation to do so. Disclosures of HIV infection by parents to children are inhibited by fears of rejection and by the desire to protect the children. The potential costs of self-disclosure are therefore pitted against the benefits of gaining support.

Opportunities to reciprocate support are another important dimension to feeling supported. Providing social support can buffer stress to an even greater extent than receiving support. For example, reciprocity decreases hostility and depression among some people with HIV infection. Many people with HIV infection seek opportunities to support others by joining support groups or volunteer organisations. The rewards of helping others with HIV infection have been reported in surveys of AIDS service volunteers. Various sources of loss associated with HIV infection, including unemployment, rejection and deaths of friends attenuate social support by shrinking the size of social networks. Illness and death of relationship partners, friends and acquaintances constrict social contacts and therefore reduce opportunities to gain and reciprocate support.

Among population subgroups hit hardest by AIDS, relationship losses have been devastating. Entire branches of gay communities have been lost, resulting in a depletion of available support for individuals with HIV infection. Paradoxically, by becoming connected to a supportive network, such as through a service organisation, an activist group, or a support group, a person increases their risk of losing relationships and constricting support that they have come to rely on.

Relationships with committed partners, friends, peers, family members and professional helpers form a structure and context of social support. Ethnic, cultural and gender differences in social networks and social stigmas in HIV infection, create barriers to support, increasing isolation among people who most need support. To gain support and opportunities to reciprocate, HIV-positive individuals must overcome barriers and selectively self-disclose. Although numbers and frequencies of social contacts are related to the availability of support, the content of relationships and the actions of others determine the support that a person receives.

Feeling supported is determined by more than mere social contact. Social interactions must address the demands of stressors if they are going to protect against emotional distress. Theories of social support traditionally encompass three functions that buffer stress and promote psychological well-being: emotional, informational and instrumental support.

Emotional support consists of affection, comforting and encouragement that result in positive effects on self-esteem feelings of self-worth and a sense of belonging. Informational support, such as advice or updated knowledge, may help people interpret, comprehend, or cope with HIV infection. Finally, materials, assistance and services have practical functions and constitute an instrumental dimension of support. All three types of support are known to promote psychological adjustment among HIV-positive individuals.

Relationships can establish and maintain emotional balance and are therefore considered a high priority in coping with HIV. Emotional support, like emotion-focused coping, does not directly address matters that affect HIV progression or the symptoms of HIV infection. Emotional support does, however, enhance psychological well-being by building hope and optimism.

Uncertainties of HIV infection can cause a strong need for information. Accurate information can lead to realistic expectations about the course of illness, which may in turn facilitate psychological adjustment. Gathering information contributes to a sense of control and problem-focused coping. The value of informational support has led to a proliferation of information networks and newsletters about HIV and AIDS. It is important to note that denial can interfere with the potential benefits of informational support by blocking interest and openness to information.

Practical assistance with everyday needs helps to reduce distress and increase positive health appraisals. In some circumstances, instrumental support can have greater psychological benefits in HIV infection than either emotional or informational support. The availability of assistance can relieve stress caused by physical limitations. As has been the case with other psychological dimensions of HIV infection, the need for and availability of instrumental support, as well as other types of social support, changes over the course of HIV infection.

After initially testing HIV positive, individuals tend to be in crisis and benefit most from strong emotional and informational supports, which are unfortunately often unavailable because of fears, stigmas and attitudes toward sickness, death and AIDS. Initial responses from post-HIV antibody test counsellors and AIDS service organisations usually offer assistance when there are few other sources. After the initial receipt of test results and as HIV infection progresses, the need for multiple types of support from multiple sources increases. Fatigue, diminished self-esteem, physical disability and illness reduce an individual's ability to maintain interpersonal relationships.

Illness therefore brings dissatisfaction with support even when it is available. Hays et al. found that satisfaction with informational support affected psychological adjustment but depended on the number of HIV symptoms a person had. Gay men with more symptoms and less informational support were most depressed in relation to men with few symptoms and high informational support. Thus, informational support appeared to buffer the stress associated with developing symptoms.

Relationships between social support and illness suggest that individuals who are most in need of support are therefore inclined to be dissatisfied with the support that they receive. Decreased availability of social support at later phases of HIV infection contributes to anger, resentment, hopelessness and depression. HIV infection invariably leads to hospitalisations, disabilities, unemployment and fatigue, all of which contribute to social isolation. People in one's support networks may die from AIDS, others become emotionally exhausted and still others turn away from sickness and anticipatory loss.

People with AIDS therefore seek support from multiple sources, particularly when compared with their asymptomatic HIV-positive and HIV-negative counterparts (Hays). Attempting to meet increased needs for support, AIDS service organisations, mental health and medical providers and others have derived a host of social support interventions modelled after programs for other chronic and life-threatening illnesses.

Social support interventions

Interventions for individuals affected by the HIV epidemic provide emotional, informational and instrumental support. The most organised and accessible interventions have thus far included support groups, volunteer programs and hospice services.

Support groups for people with HIV infection and their caregivers are similar to those for other medical patients. Groups have been used to foster interpersonal relationships that benefit people with HIV infection and those who provide their care. To date, there has been only one published clinical trial that tested different models of support for HIV-positive therapy clients.

Kelly, Murphy, Bahr, Kalichman, et al. randomly assigned 68 HIV-positive (non-AIDS) men with heightened depressed mood to one of three experimental treatment conditions: a cognitive-behavioural treatment group, a social support group and an individual psychotherapy comparison condition. Kelly, Murphy, Bahr, Kalichman, *et al.* described the cognitive-behavioural condition as follows:

> The cognitive-behavioural groups focused on the use of cognitive and behaviour strategies to reduce maladaptive anxiety and depression.

In describing the social support group condition, Kelly, Murphy, Bahr, Kalichman, et al. stated that

> the support group condition was modelled after the type of social support groups commonly used in coping with other types of illness (such as cancer) and often offered to HIV-positive persons by community AIDS service programs. Leaders of the support groups encouraged members to describe their feelings about having HIV infection; to identify shared problems, concerns, fears and hopes; to discuss how these issues are handled; and to adopt supportive and encouraging roles toward others in the group. There was considerable member-initiated discussion of how problems related to HIV were handled and participants were encouraged to share with and learn from, experiences raised by others in the group. The group members generated the discussion topics of each session. Members often chose to talk generally about how it felt to have the group as a place to share with others their concerns about HIV. Skills training, behaviour rehearsal, contracting and practice assignments were not employed in this condition.

Results of the study showed that both support group models positively affected group members relative to the control group. However, the social support group appeared to have the greatest benefit over a 3-month follow-up period. Eighty-six percent of the social support group participants demonstrated clinically significant improvement on an index of distress severity, whereas two thirds of the comparison condition showed clinical deterioration, regressing below baseline levels during 3 months.

Although members of the cognitive-behavioural group demonstrated a pattern of clinical change that was intermediate between the social support group and the control condition, cognitive-behavioural group participants did decrease their use of illicit substances to a greater degree than the other two groups. Kelly, Murphy, Bahr, Kalichman, et al. concluded that the two group models provided different types of support with different outcomes. Whereas the social support group allowed more time for emotional support and therefore emotion-focused coping, the cognitive-behavioural group emphasized problem-focused and active coping skills training.

Thus, emotional adjustment was greatest among the social support group members, whereas declines in maladaptive coping behaviours occurred among the skills training participants. Curiously, decreased illicit drug use did not seem to correspond to reductions in distress. These findings highlight the differential effects of emotional and informational support groups for people adjusting to HIV infection.

Support groups can help people with HIV infection achieve a sense of emotional balance. Emotion-focused support groups emphasize hope, opportunities to gain insights from others, emotional catharsis and interpersonal connectedness. Mathews and Bowes identified several dimensions of effective HIV-related support groups, including sharing common experiences, group cohesiveness, reinforcing hope, helping others and learning from others' experiences.

Sadovsky suggested that support groups deal with a client's fears and prejudices, coordinate community services, encourage independence and hope, allow for focusing on self and promote informed choices. HIV-related support groups can facilitate emotional expression, promote acceptance and reduce illness-related fears. Bringing people with comparable life situations together creates a potentially supportive environment through a sense of mutual understanding. Support groups also provide opportunities to deal with immediate crises.

Psychosocial problem solving often occurs naturally in support groups. The goals of another support group described in the literature were to provide an environment for exchanging coping strategies and reinforcing health management behaviours. Support groups allow for the sharing of concerns among peers and serve as a vehicle for developing and reinforcing coping strategies. However, for many people, support groups are most productive when they have tangible outcomes, such as when new friendships are formed or when new information is gained.

Support groups can include information dissemination pertinent to HIV infection and treatment. Alternatively, groups can focus exclusively on delivering and exchanging information, providing a forum for people with HIV infection to share experiences, knowledge and ideas. Knowledgeable group facilitators can become a primary source of information. Expert speakers may also be invited to provide specialised information to group members, including infectious disease physicians, pharmacists, nutritionists, insurance agents, social welfare workers and so on.

There are several examples of information-based support groups. Coleman and Harris conducted a psychoeducational support group to meet five specific information needs: information pertaining to HIV disease; management of health problems; health care and health insurance concerns; nutrition and its role in HIV infection; and issues of sexuality and intimate relationships.

Similarly, Hedge and Glover described an informational support group that focused on general health, stress, diet, medications, the medical system, legal issues, relationships, safer sex, complementary therapies and life-style changes brought about by HIV infection. The information content of sessions and the information needs of group members vary during the course of HIV infection. In the context of a support group, people receive information along with emotional support, as well as have the chance to share information with others, therefore reciprocating support.

Support groups vary widely in structure and format. Groups may have limited numbers of sessions or go on indefinitely. Groups can have a set agenda or evolve over time. Support groups may be open with regard to allowing in new members, or closed to new members for the life of the group. Formatting groups as either open or closed requires choosing between the benefits of fresh perspectives in open groups or the benefits of trust and confidentiality fostered by closed groups.

Another issue is group composition. Mixing clients who recently tested HIV positive with those who have been HIV positive for a long time, versus limiting groups to individuals at a particular phase of HIV infection, affects the issues addressed by the group. Certain types of support are needed after initial diagnosis compared with during symptomatic illness. Including recently diagnosed people and long-term survivors in the same group allows the newly diagnosed to gain emotional and informational support from those who have "been there" and survived HIV infection.

On the other hand, the newly diagnosed can become distressed when confronted by AIDS. Decisions regarding group composition therefore shape many of the issues that arise in sessions. Other decisions include whether to mix groups or keep them homogeneous with respect to gender, sexual orientation and modes of having contracted HIV infection. Although homogenous groups are often considered more effective, there are benefits to diversity.

Professional versus peer facilitators, co-facilitators versus a single facilitator, whether to invite outside speakers and the degree to which group members and facilitators should be matched for sexes, ethnicity and HIV status are issues that require careful consideration. Unfortunately, there have been few empirical studies to guide these decisions. One study reported interviews that focused on the experiences and perceptions of support groups for people with HIV infection. All of the interview participants who had known they were HIV positive for more than a few months had attended at least one support group offered by AIDS service organisations.

It was almost universal that the emotional tone of support groups influenced participant satisfaction. Most desired groups focused on positive attitudes and hope, rather than expression of negative feelings and sharing the perils of HIV infection. Information exchange was another critical factor in the perceived effectiveness of support groups. Information, including that shared by fellow support group members, was considered among the greatest benefits.

Emotional support is gained from the feeling of not being alone. Groups can foster friendships and opportunities for activities or social events.

With respect to group composition, Kalichman found that the majority of gay men and heterosexual women felt comfortable coming to a mixed group and believed that diversity facilitated support. However, heterosexual men and injection drug users felt that their issues were different from those of gay men and heterosexual women and preferred separate groups. Perceptions of mixing different phases of HIV infection depended on stage of illness.

Those early in the course of HIV infection felt that they could benefit from the experience of people who had been HIV positive longer. For example, one man who had been HIV positive for 5 years stated, "There is a lot of support in seeing someone who has survived a long time with HIV and hear their stories." On the other hand, those at later phases believed that the newly diagnosed could offer emotional support and encouragement, but to a lesser degree than other long-term survivors.

Groups can meet the support needs of caregivers and people bereaved from AIDS. Caregiver support groups afford the opportunity to reflect, express and reconcile feelings related to caring for the ill. Support groups for caregivers are therefore geared toward sustaining emotional well-being to enable caregivers to continue their care. Like groups for people with HIV infection, caregiver support groups require addressing multiple losses. Helping people with HIV infection means repeated exposure to death and dying.

The death of a person to AIDS results in bereavement similar to that found in loss from other chronic illnesses. Support groups assist survivors in rebuilding their lives. The need for support during bereavement is well recognised. Lennon et al. found that grief reactions were greatest among those who had cared for a friend dying of AIDS who did not have their own support system.

In addition, 31 per cent of the men in the Lennon et al. study indicated that they did not receive adequate instrumental support when providing care for their friend and were not receiving emotional support while grieving. There have been few systematic studies of support groups for individuals who have suffered AIDS-related losses. In one small study, three men and four women who suffered a personal loss because of AIDS participated in a support group based on cognitive and behavioural coping strategies.

AIDS service organisations that provide support to people with HIV infection rely on volunteers, many of whom are HIV-positive themselves. For example, programs may designate a buddy to provide one-to-one support for a person with HIV infection. Buddy volunteer programs provide both companionship and physical assistance. Volunteers visit and telephone others with HIV infection as well as provide instrumental support by shopping, cleaning, cooking and transportation.

When individuals with HIV infection themselves volunteer to help others, they have the opportunity to gain support from a network of fellow volunteers as well as the reciprocity of support offered by these relationships. Volunteer experiences can increase self-esteem, enhance personal worth and give a sense of meaning.

Hospice is an interdisciplinary approach to caring for patients with terminal illnesses, where recovery is unlikely and a prognosis is stated in months or weeks. Hospice care emphasizes the quality rather than quantity of life, holistic approaches to pain control that include psychological and spiritual pain and the involvement of family and others in the care of the patient. Hospice care also supports caregivers; by providing respite and convalescent care.

Another important aspect of hospice is its emphasis on palliative care. Palliation is a specialised form of care for patients with advanced progressive diseases where curative treatments are no longer feasible. Thus, hospice care integrates psychological, social and medical approaches to address the multidimensional issues of the terminally ill. The progressive and terminal nature of HIV infection places it within the scope of the hospice mission. Unfortunately, many traditional hospices have been unwilling to accept AIDS patients into their services. The reluctance to care for people with AIDS has primarily been because of conflicts between aspects of HIV disease and eligibility criteria for hospice care.

For example, people with AIDS often do not have a family member or friend willing to be designated as a primary caregiver, a necessity for hospice home care. Moreover, AIDS has a largely unpredictable course, with sudden changes and reversals of life-threatening conditions. Additional problems may occur in relation to characteristics of certain AIDS patients, such as the continued use of illicit drugs. These aspects of AIDS set the disease apart from other chronic illnesses serviced by most hospice agencies. Thus, hospices have been started to exclusively care for people with AIDS.

In general, the same hospice care is delivered, including an emphasis on pain control and quality of life, while also offering specialised care for AIDS. The same may be said for other psychosocial interventions, where the structure and mechanisms of care are not altered but the therapeutic context and treatment are tailored to address AIDS-related needs.

Selected Readings

Campbell, C. A. (1990), Prostitution and AIDS. In D. G. Ostrow (ed.), *Behavioural aspects of AIDS.* New York: Plenum Press.

Catania, J. A., Turner, H. A., Choi, K., & Coates, T. J. (1992). "Coping with death anxiety: Help-seeking and social support among gay men with various HIV diagnoses". *AIDS.*

Cockerell, C. J. (1992), Cutaneous and historic signs of HIV infection other than Kaposi's sarcoma. In G. P. Wormser (ed.), *AIDS and other manifestations of HIV infection.* New York: Raven Press.

Finley, J. L., Joshi, V. V., & Neil, J. S. A. (1992), General pathology of HIV infection. In G. P. Wormser (ed.) *AIDS and other manifestations of HIV infection.* New York: Raven Press.

Fischl, M. A. (1992), Treatment of HIV infection. In M. A. Sande & P. A. Volberding (eds.), *The medical management of AIDS.* Philadelphia: Saunders.

Fox, R., Odaka, N., Brookmeyer, R., & Polk, B. F. (1987), "Effect of HIV antibody disclosure on subsequent sexual activity in homosexual men". *AIDS.*

Gochros, H. L. (1992), "The sexuality of gay men with HIV infection". *Social Work.*

Gupta, S., Anderson, R., & May, R. (1989), "Networks of sexual contacts: Implications for the pattern of Spread of HIV". *AIDS.*

Hackl, K., Kalichman, S. C., & Somlai, A. (1995, February). *Women with HIV/AIDS: The dual challenges of patient and primary caregiver.* Conference on HIV infection in Women, Washington, DC.

House, J. S., Landis, K. R., & Umberson, D. (1988), "Social relationships and health". *Science.*

Jillson-Boostorm, I. (1992), The impact of HIV on minority populations. In P.I. Ahmed & N. Ahmed (Eds.), *Living and dying with AIDS.* New York: Plenum Press.

5

AIDS and Environmental Stressors

The context of the HIV epidemic plays a direct role in the psychological adjustment of people who test HIV positive. Physical deterioration and uncertainties about the future make the psychological adjustment to HIV infection similar to reactions to other chronic illnesses such as cancer and heart disease. HIV infection does, however, have aspects that do not overlap with other life-threatening diseases.

HIV infection is the result of an identified virus that is contracted by socially stigmatised behaviours. AIDS is a chronic disease of the young, causing physical decline and social losses that are usually not encountered until older ages. HIV-infection-related stressors come from three primary sources: the physically debilitating effects of the disease, social losses and limitations and pre-existing problems in groups most affected by AIDS. This chapter overviews the stressors associated with HIV infection and AIDS. Here stressors refer to environmental events, situations and circumstances that commonly result in psychological distress.

Psychological adjustment to HIV infection consists of complex interactions among events, interpretations, reactions and coping resources. The focus of this chapter is on three aspects of stress: HIV-related stressors, social pressures and potential adverse effects of stress on health. Psychosocial stressors associated with HIV infection can include a history of engaging in stigmatised behaviour, long periods of asymptomatic illness and loss of physical functioning at a young age.

HIV-related stressors change over the course of the HIV infection and include HIV risk, HIV antibody testing, receiving positive antibody test results, asymptomatic HIV infection, early symptoms of illness and developing AIDS. People living in areas with high rates of AIDS experience epidemic-related stressors. Personal perceptions of risk and vulnerability are influenced by the likelihood of knowing someone with AIDS, mass media messages and the ongoing spread of HIV.

People who engage in risk behaviours in cities with high rates of AIDS can excessively worry and even become preoccupied with physical sensations perceived as symptoms. When healthy people become concerned over risk for HIV infection on the basis of their previous sexual and drug use behaviours, they can be characterised as the "worried well".

Past experiences unrelated to actual risk can lead to irrational or even phobic responses. AIDS phobia occurs most frequently among people who lack accurate information about HIV transmission and overestimate their personal risk. For example, learning that one's employee is HIV positive, getting a tattoo, or discovering that a friend has AIDS can cause unnecessary worry about having contracted HIV infection overestimating personal risk for low-probability threats is a well-known phenomenon in the risk perception literature.

Increased vividness of low-probability events makes them more imaginable and salient and therefore increases their perceived threat. For this reason, rare circumstances of HIV transmission that are widely publicised, such as contracting HIV from a dentist, are often perceived as high risk. Misinformation that was prevalent early in the HIV epidemic persists in the public's AIDS knowledge base. Media coverage and popular books based on inaccurate information have reinforced the perception that HIV is a gay disease and that HIV can be contracted through casual contacts. Dispelling myths over the course of the epidemic has taken place slowly, but some segments of the population remain unaware of basic facts about HIV and AIDS. People with established risk behaviour histories do not necessarily perceive themselves at risk for HIV infection and therefore do not experience their behaviour as a stressors.

The relationship among past behaviour, risk perceptions and sense of personal threat interacts with certain life circumstances. Personal risk perceptions are also based on identification with a known risk group as well as having engaged in risk behaviours.

A survey in Chicago showed that women of colour at high behavioural risk for HIV infection expressed relatively little concern over personal risk for HIV infection. That ethnic minority women at high behavioural risk are not overly concerned about AIDS and misperceive personal risk is particularly alarming because of the disproportionately high rates of AIDS among women of colour.

A particularly important social dimension known to affect risk perceptions is having personally known an HIV-positive person. Identification with a person who has HIV infection brings close to home the possibility of risk. In fact, identification with an HIV-infected person increases perceptions of personal risk and vulnerability. This was illustrated by the disclosure of HIV infection by basketball star Earvin "Magic" Johnson, which had an immediate and substantial impact on HIV risk perceptions among several populations, but particularly among African American men. The effects of Magic Johnson's announcement on risk perceptions were, however, relatively short-lived, with changes in perceptions running parallel to the amount of mass media coverage of the event.

Risk-related stressors influence continued risk behaviours. People living under stressful conditions engage in an array of poor health practices that ultimately result in increased risk for disease. Of particular relevance to AIDS is how stressful situations may increase rates of sexual behaviour and drug use. Perceived threat of social stressors, including crime, drug abuse and discrimination, is associated with increased frequencies of HIV risk behaviours among men and women. J. Joseph et al. found that homosexual and bisexual men with greater self-perceived risk for infection reported fewer reductions in high-risk sexual practices. Personal efforts to reduce risk for HIV infection can become stressful in and of themselves. Pressure to initiate and maintain safer sexual and drug-use behaviours and doubts that such efforts are effective, can become stressful. D. Martin found that perceptions of threat, to oneself or to others, increase efforts among gay men to reduce their risk.

Similarly, uncertainty about having contracted HIV motivates some people to seek HIV antibody testing. People who believe they are not HIV infected before seeking testing and who in fact do test negative, experience substantial relief after receiving test results.

People who do not seek testing until they have symptoms of infection, which may constitute as many as 40 per cent of individuals who test HIV antibody positive, also experience a sense of relief following the knowledge of their positive HIV status. As is the case for other life-threatening diseases, seeking pre-symptomatic testing will, if nothing else, end the stress caused by uncertainties.

HIV Antibody testing

Testing for HIV antibodies involves the possibility of learning that one has a chronic, incurable, life-threatening illness. Huggins et al. pointed out the importance of a self-assessment of personal risk for HIV infection as testing decisions. Self-assessments of HIV risk, however, are meaningless unless conducted with accurate knowledge about HIV transmission. After an informed and complete risk assessment, a person should identify their coping resources, social supports and relative coping strengths and weaknesses and develop a coping plan should their HIV antibody test result be positive.

HIV testing is offered by private physicians and medical clinics, public health clinics and community-based organisations. Testing by private providers and many public testing programs is usually confidential.

Confidential testing, however, is very different from anonymous HIV testing. In confidential testing, identifying information is obtained and kept as part of a medical record, whereas in anonymous testing, names and other identifying information are not recorded and test results are obtained through a randomly assigned numbering system. Receiving a positive HIV test result can lead to adverse social consequences, so anonymous testing offers a number of advantages.

Concerns that HIV testing is not truly anonymous are a common reason for individuals at risk to avoid testing. Despite the important distinction between confidential and anonymous testing, one study found that more than half of patients of a public sexually transmitted disease clinic did not know the difference between testing options. There are several reasons that people who perceive themselves to be at high risk for HIV infection seek testing and there are as many reasons why testing is avoided.

Siegel et al. interviewed 120 gay men and found that HIV testing was believed to provide access to medical treatments effective in combating HIV infection. They also found that men believed testing would motivate them to make positive health and life-style changes, such as reducing substance use and increasing health consciousness. Similarly, many of the men in this study reported that testing for HIV would allow them to make more informed decisions regarding sexual relationships. Some men were motivated to get tested in order to diagnose the origin of an ambiguous health condition that they feared could be related to HIV infection. Finally, they found that a substantial number of gay men got tested to relieve the psychological tension caused by not knowing their HIV antibody status.

These results, however, may not generalise to women and similar studies with women have not been conducted. Heterosexual men and women surveyed at a sexually transmitted disease clinic and gay and bisexual men surveyed in Canada appeared to engage in a cost-benefit analysis in their HIV-test decision making.

Potential for health care and relief of tension were among the most important benefits associated with HIV testing and fear of not being able to cope with a positive test result was among the most salient costs. Because of the potential benefits of testing and the emphasis on social responsibility, HIV antibody testing has become the norm in many areas with high rates of AIDS. Most high-HIV areas have accepted that testing is the healthy, ethical and informed course of action.

People who do not feel psychologically prepared to get tested, or for whatever other reason do not seek testing, may therefore be pressured to get tested. The potential benefits of HIV testing, although accepted by many, can be offset by perceived costs. Even with anonymous testing, unwanted disclosure of HIV test results is a pervasive concern among individuals who have been at risk for HIV infection. Studies have shown that a sizeable number of people at risk for HIV infection have not been tested.

A study conducted in Los Angeles county found that 37 per cent of individuals at risk for HIV infection either had not been tested or did not return for their test results. Similarly, a national survey found that 40 per cent of homosexually active men, 54 per cent of injection drug users and 67 per cent of heterosexuals at risk for HIV infection had not been tested. Perceptions of personal risk, fears of not being able to cope with infection and concerns about being socially sanctioned for testing HIV positive, all exert chilling effects on testing decisions. HIV testing shares several features in common with medical screening for other life-threatening illness like Camer and Huntington's disease among others.

For people who perceive themselves at risk for HIV infection, there are many fears that inhibit getting tested. Seeking HIV testing, regardless of the result, can affiliate a person with a risk group and have adverse social consequences. Another stressor associated with testing is the waiting period for test results, which lasts about two to three weeks. Worries and concerns escalate during the wait for test results.

Negative HIV test results usually bring relief, but they can also have adverse reactions. Individuals who test HIV negative experience pressures to modify risk behaviours.

There may also be guilt associated with having been at high risk and "gotten away with it". Finally, the perceived threat of AIDS and the lack of effective treatments cause stress among persons at risk even after testing HIV negative.

Receiving a positive HIV test result

Initial reactions to receiving positive HIV test results can be characterised by shock and denial. Receiving an HIV-positive result makes it nearly impossible for people to retain information provided to them during post-test counselling. This too parallels experiences of receiving diagnoses of other life-threatening illnesses.

HIV-positive women who have children also become immediately concerned about the possibility of their children being infected. Shortly after the immediate shock, a series of negative emotional states follow, including anger, anxiety and reactive depression.

Preoccupations with one's own mortality are also common among people who test HIV positive, further increasing their sense of vulnerability to disease and death. Receiving HIV-positive test results can lead to obsessive and compulsive health concerns, as well as anxiety specifically related to developing AIDS.

Changes in risky sexual practices occur to protect sexual partners as well as because of declines in sexual interest. However, sexual behaviour changes are not universal among people who test HIV positive. Although fear of progressing to AIDS can occur over long periods of time following receipt of positive test results, some HIV-positive persons quickly adjust. Strategies for coping are often effective following a brief period of immediate psychological distress.

In a prospective study of people at risk for HIV infection, Perry, Jacobsberg, Fishman, Weiler, et al. assessed psychological distress before, immediately after and at two weeks and ten weeks following receipt of test results. Using visual analogue scales of affective disturbance where participants reported anxiety and fears along a continuum, the study showed that people who tested HIV positive were distressed immediately before and immediately after receiving their test results.

However, distress levels significantly decreased two weeks and ten weeks later. Concerns of having infected others with HIV and fears of developing AIDS, which were also high when receiving test results, decreased at the follow-up assessments. Ironson et al. reported similar findings. Psychological adjustment has also been reported among women who tested HIV positive in the U.S. Air Force. These women were, however, not representative of women with HIV infection because they did not reside in an inner city and were of middle income. People experience psychological distress following after learning that they are HIV positive and psychological adjustment usually occurs within weeks following notification of a positive test. The traumatic impact of a life-threatening medical diagnosis is often followed by an existential plight that has subtle psychological affects.

Reactions to a positive test are influenced by the manner in which results are delivered. One study found that 23 per cent of people who test HIV positive view the delivery of results as unclear, insensitive and unkind. Adverse responses to the quality of communication during test notification are directly related to psychological distress.

The psychological effects of HIV-positive results also depend on where a person is in the HIV disease spectrum. People who test HIV positive early in the disease and in the absence of clinical symptoms become concerned about the possibility of developing symptoms and of someday having AIDS.

The situation, however, is quite different for people who wait to get tested until symptoms occur. Beevor and Catalan found that although women who test HIV negative are most likely motivated to get tested by their past behaviours, women who test positive are motivated by HIV-related symptoms.

News of being infected with HIV when already symptomatic shortens the time line for developing AIDS and in some cases notification of HIV infection occurs simultaneously with an AIDS diagnosis. Thus, delay of testing until symptoms develop complicates coping because the disease has progressed toward its later stages.

Illness-related stressors

HIV infection is a lifelong condition that results in physical decline and a very high mortality rate. People must face threats to long-term survival, the necessity of immediate lifestyle changes, fears of potentially infecting others, health concerns, changes in appearance and declining quality of life. HIV infection invariably involves a pervasive uncertainty about when HIV-related illnesses will occur.

Uncertainty is exacerbated by long asymptomatic periods permeated by illnesses. Symptoms appear and disappear, keeping patients on constant watch. Coupled with uncertainties about disease progression is the loss of control over directing one's own future. People who test HIV-positive know that a debilitating and life-threatening illness may strike at any time, causing the stress of a "walking time bomb". Long asymptomatic periods are eventually followed by symptomatic illnesses. During symptomatic HIV infection, almost any sign of illness an elevate anxiety. Distress, however, depends on where an individual is located on the spectrum of HIV disease.

Close monitoring of fluctuations in T-helper lymphocytes often follows awareness of being HIV positive. Early symptoms serve as a reminder that HIV disease is derading the immune system and that the virus is becoming increasingly threatening. For women with children, symptoms have the added burden of demanding assistance with child care. The onset of AIDS-related conditions causes acute distress and preacupations with illness. In a study of HIV-positive gay men who were asymptomatic, had early symptoms, or had been diagnosed with AIDS, Chuang et al. found that all three groups demonstrated substantial distress.

A seven year longitudinal study of gay and bisexual men in New York City found that knowledge of HIV seropositivity and symptoms were consistently related to psychological distress, including depression, traumatic stress reactions, suicidal ideations and increased use of sedatives.

HIV-related psychological distress also occurs in response to concerns over medical treatments aimed at controlling HIV infection. Multiple hospitalisations, intrusive treatments, the threat of side effects and uncertainty over treatment effectiveness are also common occurrences.

The need for medications, usually in large amounts taken several times a day, can continually disrupt attempts to cope with HIV infection. Contributing further to distress associated with treatments is that they are taken without the potential for a cure. AIDS is like cancer with respect to its life-threatening nature, lifelong ration, illness concerns and existential issues.

Like cancer, HIV infection is related to physical decline, bodily disfigurement, loss of physical functioning, emotional anguish, financial crisis, pain and death. Both diseases are also catastrophic. People with HIV infection can therefore have psychological reactions characteristic of stress responses.

The course of cancer and other life-threatening diseases, however, includes the availability of multiple curative treatments.

Thus, psychological adjustment to a life-threatening disease relies heavily on the degree to which there are real possibilities for cure. In contrast with cancer, it is not possible to offer curative attempts for HIV infection. The clinical course of HIV infection is therefore significantly different from that of other diseases.

Although HIV-related illnesses are treated and lives are extended, illness signifies the underlying disease. Symptomatic illness can be treated until, ultimately, there are no treatment responses and death ensues. The prospect of persistent opportunistic illnesses in the midst of a degenerating immune system therefore poses a relentless succession of psychological challenges.

SOCIAL STRESSORS

Knowledge that one has HIV infection necessarily alters the nature of close interpersonal relationships. Being HIV positive can bring about fears of abandonment by friends and family, rejection from coworkers and loss of employment. Losses associated with AIDS can be particularly devastating because they occur out of synch with developmental expectations.

Social losses

A positive HIV antibody test result can lead to loss of employment, the threat of eviction, denial of health and life insurance, refusal of professional services denial of health and dental care. People with HIV often suffer disruptions to their partnered or intimate relationships. Sexual practices must be limited to protect sexual partners from infection, as well as to protect people with HIV from reinfection and exposure to other sexually transmitted diseases.

These issues are magnified for women with HIV, involved in power-imbalanced relationships, where control in changing sexual practices is minimal. Disclosure of HIV infection to a partner for his or her protection may even place women at risk for violent repercussions. Individuals with HIV infection must decide how and when to disclose their HIV status to sexual partners.

Disclosure of HIV-positive status to sexual partners can lead to rejection because of fears, inability to cope, not being able to deal with the potential loss of a partner and dissatisfaction with new limitations placed on the relationship. Fears of losing a partner at a time when support is most needed may inhibit disclosing serostatus altogether.

Losses associated with HIV infection-AIDS and their causes

- *Employment:* due to infection status or disability
- *Family:* fears and stigmas or inability to cope
- *Friends:* fears and stigmas, inability to cope, or friends dying of AIDS
- *Health care:* inability to obtain insurance benefits
- *Financial:* health-care costs coupled with diminished employment
- *Social supports:* fears and stigmas or inability to cope
- *Self-esteem and pride:* self-blame for the epidemic and personal infection

- *Physical/affectionate contact:* irrational fears of casual transmission
- *Future goals and aspirations:* facing a chronic life-threatening illness
- *Sexual partners:* fears or inability to cope
- *Physical functioning:* disease progression
- *Pets:* potential to carry pathogens
- *Life-style changes:* potential ill effects on health, such as smoking and alcohol

Disclosure of HIV infection is usually a selective process. Huggins et al. showed that HIV-infected gay men tend to disclose their serostatus to sexual partners they felt emotionally invested in, as opposed to more casual sexual partners. The study found that 96 per cent of men told exclusive and long-term sexual partners that they were HIV-positive, whereas only 44 per cent disclosed to regular but not exclusive partners and none disclosed to casual and anonymous sexual partners. Selective disclosure was also demonstrated in a study of HIV-positive Hispanic men.

It should be noted, however, that people who do not disclose their positive serostatus to sexual partners do not necessarily put their partners at risk, because they may alter their behaviour to protect them. Issues of informing sexual partners can be circumvented by effectively removing risks for HIV transmission. Taking responsibility to protect sexual partners from HIV infection, whether disclosure of a positive serostatus occurs or not, weighs heavily on people living with HIV. Not surprisingly, people who learn they are HIV-positive often experience conflicts and break-ups in their intimate relationships.

Bereavement

The most common source of loss for many HIV-positive people is the death of partners and friends because of AIDS. Studies have found complex interactions among cognitive, affective and behavioural reactions to the loss of someone to AIDS. Cities with high AIDS prevalence rates lose many young citizens. Thus far, multiple bereavements resulting from AIDS-related deaths have been recognised mostly among gay men. In a large Chicago cohort studied relatively early in the epidemic, 45 per cent of gay men reported knowing someone with AIDS and 35 per cent knew someone who had died of AIDS.

In a cohort of over 700 gay men in New York City who were asymptomatic for HIV-related illnesses, 27 per cent had lost a sexual partner or close friend to AIDS. Among those classified as bereaved, 18 per cent lost two and 15 per cent lost three or more persons to AIDS. When Martin included men who lost any friends to AIDS, 52 per cent of the cohort was considered bereaved. Perry, Fishman, Jacobsberg and Frances also found 55 per cent of people with HIV infection in New York City to have suffered the death of someone because of AIDS. Although multiple losses occur frequently in high-AIDS incidence areas, men who are HIV infected themselves suffer the greatest number of AIDS-related losses. HIV-positive social networks often originate in clinics, service organisations, social activities and supportive services. The fact that HIV is spread most rapidly within social-sexual networks also increases the likelihood of social connections among HIV-positive persons.

Bereavement is a well-known, multidimensional source of stress and multiple losses have additive effects. J. L. Martin described a close response relationship between the number of bereavements from AIDS a person suffers and the degree to which they experience psychological trauma. Martin observed demoralisation, sleep disruptions, affective disturbances, intrusive thoughts illicit and prescription drug use that increased proportionally with the number of AIDS-related deaths. J. L. Martin and Dean identified persistent psychological distress among both HIV-positive and HIV-negative gay men.

Men who lost someone to AIDS at any point in the 7-year study showed the greatest traumatic stress and distress symptoms increased in conjunction with the number of losses suffered. Similar results were reported by Neugebauer *et al.*, finding an increased number of bereavement symptoms, such as preoccupation with and searching for the deceased person, with increased numbers of deaths from AIDS. Bereavement from AIDS prompts a sense of AIDS vulnerability and increases the likelihood of seeking psychological assistance to cope with AIDS-related concerns. AIDS-related bereavement in HIV-positive persons has several qualitatively different dimensions. Bereaved persons with HIV are likely to self-identify with the deceased person in terms of their own mortality and each death from AIDS exacerbates fears of developing AIDS.

Women with HIV infection are likely to suffer additional stress. Women must often contend with their own HIV infection while serving as the primary caregiver for their HIV-positive partner (not unique to women with HIV), as well as caring for their children. Obviously, having an HIV-positive child further contributes to stress levels.

A qualitative study of HIV-positive women found that caring for their children and concerns about who will care for them if she should become ill is the single most significant stressor for these women. Pregnancy for HIV-positive women requires anguishing over decisions about terminating or carrying the pregnancy to term and about whether to use antiretroviral medication that may significantly reduce the risk for perinatal transmission but with unknown side effects. Issues are often complicated by conflicting advice from family, clergy, physicians and friends.

HIV-related stress develops out of fears of contracting HIV, worries about one's own behavioural risk history, knowledge of being HIV infected, waiting and worrying through asymptomatic infection the onset of HIV-related symptoms and illnesses. Surrounding HIV stressors is a second layer of pressure that exists in the immediate social context. Misinformation, fear and worry among close friends and family, as well as employers and health-care providers, can serve as sources of stress.

Finally, the attenuation of social networks because of AIDS-related deaths causes people with HIV infection to confront the ultimate outcome of AIDS.

Beyond disease-related and relationship stressors, a third dimension of AIDS-related stress involves pre-existing characteristics of subgroups most affected by AIDS.

PRE-EXISTING SOCIAL STRESSORS

AIDS has affected people from diverse ethnic, socioeconomic and sociocultural backgrounds. It is therefore less meaningful today to discuss HIV-risk groups because any person engaging in high-risk sexual or drug use behaviour is at potential risk of infection. However, because HIV spreads most rapidly within social, sexual and drug-injecting networks, particularly early in the course of an epidemic, communities with high rates of HIV seroprevalence are at greatest risk for spread. HIV infection has thus far been concentrated among gay and bisexual men and women living in large cities.

Thus, gay men, injection drug users, ethnic minorities and other socially disadvantaged groups have been hit hardest by AIDS and these persons face other multiple life stressors. Social problems surrounding groups affected most by AIDS serve as pre-existing stressors, potentially complicating HIV infection and exacerbating distress. The sections below review the pre-existing social problems relevant to homosexually active men, persons living in inner cities where injection drug use is prevalent, hemophiliacs and adults with chronic mental illness.

Gay and bisexual men

Gay and bisexual men have long been recognised as a socially stigmatised sexual minority. It is common for families to reject homosexual members and for gay men to be victims of harassment and violence. Prejudice against gay and bisexual men has subsequently been amplified by the AIDS crisis, both from outside and within gay communities.

Social isolation of gay men now results from both homophobia and AIDS phobia. Among themselves, gay men commonly assume personal responsibility for AIDS. However, communities can splinter on the basis of beliefs about risk behaviours, such as labelling people as hustlers, cruisers and blaming them for the spread of HIV.

Stress within gay communities is further potentiated by high-risk sexual practices. Although longitudinal cohort studies show substantial reductions in high-risk sexual behaviours among gay men over the course of the HIV epidemic cross-sectional surveys outside of AIDS epidemic centers have shown higher rates of risk behaviours. Continued risky sexual practices result in personal distress for many gay men. Feelings of not being able to change also leads to heightened distress.

Independent of their risk behaviour, HIV has emerged as a major source of stress for gay men living in most urban areas. Folkman et al. found that the top five most stressful life domains for homosexual and bisexual men included illness of close friends and monitoring personal health. In a large study of self-identified gay men, D. Martin identified five dimensions using a factor analysis of a threat-perception questionnaire: threats to personal goals and aspirations for the future; personal appearance; integrity; health; and the health of friends and partners. Although many sources of stress identified by Folkman *et al.* and Martin are not caused directly by HIV, the epidemic has contributed new dimensions of stress.

Cultural and ethnic differences within gay communities may lead to additional stress for gay men of colour. Homophobic reactions are more open among ethnic minorities, allowing overt rejection. It is therefore common for ethnic minority homosexual men to report stress related to accepting their own sexual orientation.

A large number of ethnic minority homosexual men do not label themselves as gay and thereby remain disconnected from gay social networks. Ethnic minority men are less likely to access information available through gay newspapers, brochures and outreach to gay bars and organisations.

Urban communities and the inner city

More than 52 per cent of all U.S. AIDS cases have originated from 16 cities. That urban areas are most affected by HIV is not unique to this epidemic. Congested living conditions, poor health resources, poverty and relatively closed social and sexual networks all increase the potential for rapid spread of disease. People with injection-drug-using addictions are well recognised as a socially disadvantaged group. Injection drug users are generally rejected and mistrusted on the basis of their drug use alone. Stress results from socio-economic stressors that co-exist with injection drug use, social stigmas associated with drug addiction and addiction to drugs itself.

Because injecting drugs is illegal, it also requires the evasion of law enforcement, another potential chronic stressor. Drug use is often a means of psychological escape from the inner city and poverty. Drug dependence is therefore commonly related to coping deficits for managing serious life stressors. Therefore, adjustment to HIV infection may be complicated for injection drug users because of vulnerability to social and personal stressors.

Women living in inner cities constitute another special population within the epidemic. Among women with AIDS, 49 per cent were infected by injection drug use and 20 per cent through sexual behaviour with an injection-drug-using partner. Inner-city women infected with HIV are predominantly ethnic minorities and therefore face prejudices and discriminations placed on members of all three subgroups: minorities, women and people with HIV. HIV-positive women may have limited access to health care and may be unable to obtain treatment for HIV infection in a timely manner.

Another major source of stress among HIV-infected women is the possibility of becoming pregnant after infection or dealing with an existing pregnancy. Women are unlikely to have prior experience discussing HIV testing with a health-care provider and may be offered testing only after they are already pregnant. Women who learn they are HIV positive early in a pregnancy must decide whether they should terminate the pregnancy.

Studies of families with injection drug users have shown that women are most often primary caregivers. Women may be caregivers in families where their spouse is also HIV positive and they may have an HIV-positive child, making it necessary for women to balance their own care with the needs of their family. HIV-positive women with uninfected partners may be rejected, emotionally isolated and financially disconnected. Women with children are burdened with finding care for their children as they anticipate becoming ill. Many women with HIV infection are single parents and must plan for the long-term safety shelter and care of their children. The number of children and adolescents orphaned by AIDS is growing at a rapid pace, with 18,500 children orphaned by AIDS at the end of 1991 and 60,000 orphans expected by the end of 1999.

Women and men living in inner cities often lack access to resources that facilitate coping with HIV infection. People with late-stage infection tend to be unemployed and without health insurance. Even when it is available, the inner-city poor and ethnic minorities may not access health care because of a social history of discrimination.

Sociopolitical abuses of the recent past have erected barriers for many disadvantaged groups. For example, the Tuskegee Syphilis Study, funded by the U.S. federal government to observe the natural history of untreated syphilis, followed a cohort of African American men in the 1930s to 1972. In this study, syphilis was allowed to progress and partners became infected without intervention. The Tuskegee study formed the basis of an understandable distrust of public health agencies among African Americans. These barriers pose obvious problems for managing HIV infection and act as additional stressors for ethnic minorities.

Moreover, because of such events as the Tuskegee Study, ethnic minorities frequently express the belief that HIV is a means of oppression, as well as a form of genocide. The social context of AIDS, particularly in urban areas, forms a complex hierarchy of competing life stressors and survival needs, of which AIDS is one of several. In a study of women living in Chicago, Kalichman et al. examined the relationships among stress-related social problems facing urban women. The study found several life stressors perceived as more immediately pressing than AIDS, including employment, child care and crime. Kalichman et al. also found that each social problem was perceived as a more serious concern for ethnic minorities than for nonminorities.

In a follow-up study, Kalichman, Somlai, et al. (in press) conducted a similar survey of male and female patients of a sexually transmitted disease clinic, 78 per cent of whom were African American and 74 per cent of whom were living in poverty. Because the sample was drawn from a clinic, it was thought that the participants would be more sensitised to AIDS than a general community sample.

Men and women rated 11 social problems along dimensions of perceived seriousness. Results replicated Kalichman *et al.*'s findings by showing that AIDS was perceived as a greater concern than housing, alcoholism and child care, but less of a problem than employment, crime, discrimination, drug abuse and teen pregnancy.

Those who are HIV infected face a number of medical complications, added expenses and the compounded stress of life-threatening illnesses.

Pre-existing mental health problems

In a prospective study conducted among persons at risk for HIV infection, Perry, Jacobsberg, Fishman, Frances et al. found high prevalence rates of psychological disturbances among HIV risk groups prior to receiving their HIV test results. Lifetime rates of psychiatric syndromes were roughly two times that of epidemiologic studies; 60 per cent of men and 72 per cent of women receiving HIV testing had a history of psychological disturbances. Among those who tested HIV positive, the rates were nearly seven times as high as epidemiologic studies. High rates of psychological problems suggest substantial vulnerability to psychological distress and maladjustment for many people with HIV infection. There is also considerable overlap between characteristics of some HIV-risk groups and psychological disturbances. In particular, injection drug use is closely associated with antisocial personality disorder. Studies also suggest higher rates of bipolar affective and substance-abuse disorders among homosexually active men at risk for HIV infection.

Nearly one third of HIV-positive gay men in one study had a personality disorder diagnosis, a significantly higher rate than that found among HIV-negative gay men. Comorbidity of psychiatric history and HIV infection can complicate the course of illness by disrupting treatment and increasing hospitalisations. Recent research has focused on the HIV risk of chronic mentally ill adults. A majority of psychiatric patients are sexually active, frequently contract sexually transmitted infections and often exhibit other HIV risk behaviours. Several factors contribute to HIV risk among chronic mentally ill adults, including a lack of accurate information about HIV transmission, misperceptions of personal risk, failure to recognise risk-producing situations and difficulty communicating assertively in sexual relationships.

In addition, psychiatric patients may be particularly vulnerable to contracting HIV infection because of impulsive sexual behaviours, relationships characterised by turmoil and transiency the overlap among risk taking, psychopathology and cognitive disturbances that leads to poor judgment.

STRESS AND HEALTH

The multiple and competing pressures and demands in the lives of HIV-positive persons interfere with their quality of life. The relationship between stress and physical health among persons with HIV infection is, however, less clear. Psychoneuroimmunology, the study of central nervous system and immune system interactions, has extensively investigated the mechanisms underlying psychological influences on immune diseases. There is a substantial body of evidence that shows that both acute and chronic stressful life events affect several branches of the immune system. Negative life events and lack of social supports also increase the likelihood of illness.

Minor stressful life events may accumulate over time and act as chronic stressors, with similar effects on the immune system. The immune system reacts to chronic stress with long-term suppressed responses. The effects of stress on the immune system have therefore been widely observed, but it has not been determined if the nature and magnitude of such changes alter susceptibility to disease. Several studies have reported links among depression, immune functioning and disease, but the findings have not been conclusive. Depression that lasts days, however, can alter several branches of the immune system. Suppressed immune activity occurs as a direct result of bereavement following the death of a spouse, independent of the stress effects of caregiving. Immune disruptions are therefore observed among people who are stressed, depressed and bereaved.

The immune system is affected by stress through complex interactions among the central nervous and endocrine systems. Laboratory experiments have shown that changes in the immune system occur within 15 minutes after exposure to a mild stressor and that changes can persist for long periods of time. Perceptions of threatening situations activate the sympathetic branch of the autonomic nervous system to invoke a "flight or fight" response.

Activation of the sympathetic nervous system may directly affect the immune system through innervation of the hypothalamus and immune system organs. Hormones released during stress mediate central nervous system and immune system activities. For example, cortisol is released under stress, during depression and following periods of social deprivation. Cortisol also suppresses immune system responses, particularly with regard to reducing counts of T-helper lymphocytes. Retrospective and prospective studies have reported relationships among stressful life events, psychological distress, upper-respiratory illnesses and a number of bacterial infections. Stress is also involved in the progression of viral infections. In addition, stress affects the course of latent viral infections such as herpes simplex viruses, cytomegalovirus and Epstein-Barr virus.

There are two potential mechanisms by which stress can complicate the course of HIV infection. First, stressful events, as they have an impact on the central nervous and endocrine systems, may directly affect branches of the immune system of relevance to HIV infection. Cortisol is of particular importance because it affects the blood concentration and functions of T-helper lymphocytes. The second potential role that stress may play in HIV progression involves the activation of HIV itself. For example, Markham, Salahuddin, Veren, Orndorff and Gallo found that corticosteroids and other stress-related hormones enhance the expression and release of HIV.

Despite the evidence that stress has immunologic effects, the likelihood that stress-related reactions interact with the expression of infectious disease and the logical formulation of hypotheses that stress reactions interact with HIV disease, research has not confirmed these relationships. For example, a study of asymptomatic men with HIV infection did not find bereavement or clinical depression to significantly predict any of several markers of immune functioning. However, this study did report that for men who were not bereaved, depressive mood, although not clinical depression, was correlated with immune markers relevant to HIV disease. The authors acknowledged that these relationships may have been mediated by awareness of physical decline that may accompany both decreased immune function and depressed mood.

In another study, researchers failed to identify relationships among measures of psychological distress and immune functions in HIV infection, although an active coping style did correlate with some immune markers. Thus, some studies have suggested relationships among psychological factors and immune functions in HIV infection, but there has not been a consistent pattern of results. Research has more often failed to identify any stress-immune system relationships of clinical relevance in HIV infection.

In one study, stress-induced activation of the sympathetic nervous system did not result in loss of T-helper lymphocytes beyond that already seen in the early phases of HIV infection. A follow-up study of this sample also failed to identify relationships among distress, levels of cortisol and markers of immune system functioning. In addition, widely accepted effects of depression on immune system functioning are not observed among HIV-infected individuals. Highly stressful life events do not predict the onset of HIV-related symptoms among gay men.

Cross-sectional analyses by J. B. W. Williams, Rabkin, Remien, Gorman and Ehrhardt failed to find relationships between measures of psychological distress with markers of immune functioning in HIV-positive gay men. In a prospective study of 221 people with HIV infection not diagnosed with AIDS, Perry, Ryan, Ashman and Jacobsberg found that psychological distress was not associated with immune markers, in both concurrent and prospective analyses.

Failure to consistently identify associations between emotional reactions to stress and immune system response among people with HIV infection may be due to the pervasive damage caused by HIV. That is, immune responses in the context of HIV infection are likely different from normal immune responses. Even if stress does affect immune system functioning in HIV-positive persons, the stress-immune relationships will likely differ at various phases of HIV disease, making any such relationships far more complex than they are in normal cases.

Although proposed relationships between stress and HIV disease progression are based on studies of stress-immune interactions in the psychoneuroimmunology literature, the relatively small number of studies, their methodological limitations, underrepresentation of women and ethnic minorities and lack of positive findings precludes conclusions of stress-immune relationships in HIV infection. Thus, although stress seriously affects the quality of life for persons with HIV infection, it is not clear whether stress affects HIV disease progression.

The HIV epidemic is actually composed of multiple smaller epidemics, unfolding at various rates and patterns within subpopulations. Characteristics of the disease are distinctively different across geographic regions and subgroups. Social processes related to HIV infection result in psychological distress and potential maladjustment.

SELECTED READINGS

Antoni, M., Schneiderman, N., Klimas, N., LaPerriere, A., Ironson, G., & Fletcher, M. (1991), "Disparities in psychological, neuroendoctrine, and immunologic patterns in asymptomatic HIV-1 seropositive and seronegative gay men". *Biological Psychiatry.*

Linn, J. G., Lewis, F. M., Cain, V. A., & Kimbrough, G. A. (1993), "HIV-illness, social support, sense of coherence, and psychosocial well-being in a sample of help-seeking adults". *AIDS Education and Prevention.*

Markowitz, J. C., Klerman, G. L., & Perry, S. W. (1993), "An interpersonal psychotherapeutic approach to depressed HIV-seropositive patients". In W. H. Sledge & A. Tasman (eds.), *Clinical challenges in psychiatry.* Washington, DC: American Psychiatric Press.

Miller, D. & Riccio, M. (1990), Editorial review: Non-organic psychiatric and psychosocial syndromes associated with HIV-1 infection and disease. *AIDS.*

Naficy, A. B., & Soave, R. (1992), Cryptosporidiosis, isosporiasis, and microsporidiosis in AIDS. In G. P. Wormser (ed.), *AIDS and other manifestation of HIV infection.* New York: Raven Press.

6

Rise of Western AIDS Epidemic

A crucial error in identification would go undiscovered for years, causing confusion and hampering progress. The story of this error begins at the Institute Pasteur, where Francoise Barre-Sinoussi, Jean-Claude Chermann and Luc Montagnier found the first AIDS virus. Its activity was detected in the lymph node of a young gay man who was given the code name "Bru." He was infected but had not yet developed AIDS, a point that turned out to be very important. The Pasteur group ran into trouble when it tried to grow and isolate the virus.

The Bru lymph node was first cultured in early January 1983 and, on January 15, it shed an enzyme absolutely unique to the lentivirus group. Now called HIV- I Bru, the virus was initially called JBB/LAV. Bru's initials plus an acronym for lymphadenovirus, or lymph node virus. The Bru virus grew slowly and with difficulty, but its identity and activity were reported in the May 20, 1983, issue of Science. The Pasteur group was widely acclaimed but very worried.

In the world of virology, finding a new virus is not enough: you must propagate and isolate the organism for analysis by other virologists. The French had not yet isolated their new lentivirus and, since it proved hard to grow, they feared they might lose it. On June 26 they started a second Bru culture (JBB2/LAV). In July, Montagnier sent a sample of this second culture to Bob Gallo of the US National Cancer Institute (NCI) in Bethesda, Maryland. That same month, Chermann sent DNA from the virus to Beatrice Hahn and Flossie Wong-Staal, then working with Gallo. The virus did not thrive in Gallo's laboratory and the DNA was never analysed.

The French had found a similar virus in a man who already had AIDS. On June 9 Barre-Sinoussi began to culture this second virus, code-named "Lai." It grew much faster than Bru and also grew on permanent cell lines-cells made immortal by various techniques-whereas the Bru virus grew only on primary cells. Everybody was delighted because virologists have a prejudice for fast-growing viruses and for viruses that grow on cell lines. Viruses that grow on primary cells are much less convenient for two reasons. First, primary cells come from living donors, who must provide them every few days. Second, primary cells produce virus only temporarily because they quickly die, especially after infection with HIV.

On July 20 Barre-Sinoussi prepared to culture both Bru and Lai again. For only the first or second time, she would use new co-cultivation techniques developed in late June or early July. Designed to maintain a cell-killing virus, this protocol involved addition of growth factors and fresh activated lymphocytes at the beginning of the culture and throughout the process.

So Barre-Sinoussi collected fresh CD_4^+ cells and divided them between two flasks. Then she added a Bru sample to one flask and a Lai sample to the other. As before, Lai grew in five days, but, surprisingly, Bru grew in nine days instead of the twelve days it had previously required. Not only that, but this Bru was found later to grow in cell lines. Unfortunately, it was also found-much later-that the Lai culture had somehow contaminated the Bru culture. The Bru strain of virus grew well because it was being overtaken by the more active Lai strain. Labelled JBB2'/LAV, the mixed culture was sent for analysis to Gallo in September 1983 and to Robin Weiss, in London, in February 1984. Nobody knew it was actually Bru/Lai bearing the pseudonym of Bru.

The original Bru virus that remained at Pasteur was forgotten in a lab freezer until controversy arose, eight years later, as to who had isolated the very first HIV strain. Until then, the Bru virus, which everybody thought they were using for research and development of HIV tests, was never used by anybody for any purpose. The switch of two strains of the same virus subtype might make little difference in some cases. However, the exchange of Lai for Bru was a virological horror story. The real Bru was a much better prototype of the HIV causing the Western epidemic than was the Lai virus masquerading as Bru.

As much as one or two years before AIDS develops, the virus suddenly grows very rapidly and makes blood cells clump to form giant syncytial cells. The virus is then much more transmissible to permanent cell lines. However, many scientists believe the virus at that stage is much less transmissible among actual human beings, if only because health and sexual activity begin to decline. The virus has less chance for transmission and, if transmitted, appears more likely to be defeated by the immune defense of its new host. So a virus at the Lai stage rarely circulates and is less infectious than a virus like Bru. Virologists who were studying Lai (misnamed Bru), thriving on permanent cell lines, would have learned far more about HIV- 1 and AIDS from the real Bru, despite its culture difficulties. They were like the man in the joke, looking for his keys under a streetlight: he hadn't lost them there, but the light was good.

The fact that the HIV strains conveniently growing on cell lines had little to do with the spread of the HIV epidemic did not dawn on anyone for quite a long time. After three years, Brigitta Asjo and Eva-Maria Fenyo of the Karolinska Institute in Sweden discovered the important biological distinction between slow/low HIV and rapid/high HIV. The slow HIV is found in 95 per cent of people newly infected with the virus.

The fast HIV is found in only 5 per cent of people newly infected but in about 50 per cent of those who have progressed to AIDS. The slow/low and rapid/high designations describe HIV strains according to their speed and level of growth in culture. Unfortunately, the Asjo-Fenyo discovery was not generally known or used to unmask Lai as an imposter. So for several years we learned more than we needed to know about one virus (Lai) and nothing at all about the virus we really cared about (Bru).

The virologists' preference for strains grown on cell lines caused confusion and would lead to controversy between Gallo and Montagnier. We must now backtrack to late 1983 and early 1984, when the mixed Bru-Lai samples (mislabled JBB2/LAV) were sent to Gallo in the United States and Weiss in England. Both groups had heard that Bru was hard to grow on cell lines. However, they attempted this feat and, of course, they succeeded. What they never guessed was that, by doing this, they both simultaneously-completed the switch from Bru to Lai. In their laboratories, Lai quickly overgrew and obliterated Bru and the researchers began to propagate and study the wrong strain.

At this time the Gallo group was growing other viruses, seeking to identify the first truly US strain of HIV. This would cause problems, especially since the researchers proceeded in a strange way. On November 15, 1983, Mika Popovic pooled the cultures of various HIVs of US origin. Then on January 2, 1984, he added cultures from seven more US individuals, all from groups at high risk for AIDS. Meanwhile, he was doing work on the French virus. In February, by some miracle, he isolated Lai virus from the pooled US samples! Of course, the French culture had contaminated the US samples, "but Popovic mistook Lai for a new strain. He inoculated it onto the permanent human T-cell line H9 (Hut 78) and began producing HIV-1 Lai, which he named HIV-1 IIIB. As late as 1994, Luc Montagnier and anybody who received his virus samples was working not with HIV-A Bru but with HIV-1 Lai without knowing it. Similarly, Bob Gallo and anybody who used his virus samples was working not with HIV-1 IIIB but, again, with HIV-1 Lai. The final irony is that, not only was HIV-1 Lai going under two pseudonyms, but it never actually infected the man for whom it was named. The virus that everyone was using had undergone genetic mutations and was no longer the strain isolated at Pasteur.

It had become an unusual strain that has never infected anyone by the normal routes of HIV transmission. Except for three workers infected in the laboratory, it has infected only lab cultures. Yet this odd strain was long used to generate HIV antibodies for tests to diagnose newly infected people and monitor our blood supplies. These tests were extremely useful but were probably less sensitive than optimum. Both Montagnier and Gallo were responsible for contaminations. However, the French had the good luck to contaminate their cultures with their own virus, while the Americans had the bad luck to contaminate their cultures with someone else's virus.

Apparently, the US strains pooled by Popovic all had slow growth characteristics. They could not be adapted to cell lines, which allowed Lai to stand out. But in late 1983 the Gallo group succeeded in growing a Haitian isolate, HIV-1 RF, on a permanent cell line. In 1984, the group repeated this coup with HIV-1 MN, an isolate from a child infected in Newark, New Jersey. Then Jay Levy of the University of California, San Francisco, isolated several US strains of HIV-1 from homosexual men living in the San Francisco area. Gallo's HIV-1 MN strain from Newark would become very important. It was found among samples drawn from several children born to mothers with AIDS or at risk for AIDS. MN was born October 1980 to an IV drug-using mother. (His initials were changed to protect his identity.) When about one year old, the boy started to bleed internally due to the shortage of red blood cells that often accompanies HIV infection.

The shortage is caused mainly by destruction of red cells in the spleen so, according to common procedure, the boy's spleen was removed. This was done in 1984, when MN had yet to show any immunological abnormalities or signs of AIDS. His spleen tissue was sent to Gallo's laboratory and a virus was recovered from the cultured cells. Surprisingly, it was found to grow readily on cell lines and, unlike Lai, to resemble closely the average HIV strain circulating among infected gay men and drug users in Europe and the United States. So the virological horror story had at least one happy ending. He unwittingly replaced it with a second virus, HIV-1 Lai. Neither Gallo nor Weiss discovered the switch but instead got Montagnier's second virus to grow in cell lines.

Years later, Gallo was accused of stealing Montagnier's first virus (Bru) and claiming credit for its discovery.

But to everyone's chagrin, including his own, Gallo himself found that HIV-1 IIIB was actually Lai and bore no resemblance to the original Bru strain. (Remember, he had received the original Bru in July 1983 but could not grow it. He had received more Bru in September, but it was contaminated and ultimately overtaken by Lai.) It was Lai that Popovic succeeded in growing on permanent cell lines. It was Lai that contaminated the pooled culture from which Popovic hoped to recover the first specifically US HIV-1 strain. It was Lai that went to several pharmaceutical companies for production of HIV antibody tests. Then, in 1984, Gallo's laboratory isolated HIV-1 MN. But which of the two isolates, the French HIV-A Lai or the American HIV-1 MN, was the most typical of the virus population ravaging the Western world? The definitive answer came between 1987 and 1990, when serological and molecular methods were developed to detect the "signature" of virus strains.

A feature of the virus envelope is clearly distinctive for most strains. By comparing this feature among many strains, they found that those closely related to HIV-1 MN constituted more than 95 per cent of the viruses recovered from HIV-infected people in the United States and Europe, whether they were merely seropositive or had actually developed AIDS. Lai was not found in a single person. Montagnier and Gallo each won "first prize." The French isolated the first AIDS virus ever (HIV-1 Lai) and the Americans isolated the first virus that was truly representative of the Western AIDS epidemic (HIV-1 MN). The original Bru was even more representative, due to its slow-growing properties, but nobody—not even Montagnier—realised this virus existed until years later.

While Montagnier and Gallo were making their landmark discoveries, other researchers were tracing the history of HIV and AIDS with surprising results. Their main question was, Where was HIV-A before it emerged among gay men in the early 1980s? Before it launched this epidemic, the virus must have caused sporadic cases that went unnoticed because they were rare or seldom lethal, or both. Were these cases sufficiently puzzling that physicians had reported them in various journals? Could we pick up a trail of such reports and follow it, case by case, to discover when and where HIV was first introduced?

Since 1980, researchers have been looking for these signposts. The older literature is well indexed (if not computerised), but one cannot look up AIDS, HIV, or even immunodeficiency. One must look for cases of P carinii pneumonia (PCP) and other odd infections. The search is slow and probably incomplete, but an intriguing picture can now be pieced together. Most people assume that the AIDS epidemic originated in large US cities with extensive homosexual populations, like New York and San Francisco and then moved to European cities like Amsterdam and Copenhagen by way of American homosexuals or by European homosexuals infected in America.

However, it now looks as if the first AIDS victims were Europeans who had never been to America or encountered American homosexuals. The most compelling cases involve two sailors, one from Norway and one from England. The Norwegian sailor had travelled extensively not only in Europe but in Africa, where he could have met HIV. He was infected sometime before 1966, when he was seen with persistent enlargement of the lymph nodes. In 1971 a sample was taken that much later, using Lai reagents in the mid 1980s, showed he was seropositive for HIV. This sample and many others pivotal to the AIDS story had luckily been frozen. Using technologies available since World War II, many scientists routinely preserve intriguing sera (in a lab freezer) or cells (in liquid nitrogen) for future reference and study.

The Norwegian sailor died in April 1976 from pneumonia, dementia and other severe neurological abnormalities. He had infected his wife, who died eight months after her husband with similar signs and symptoms. A child born to the couple in 1967 developed generalised candida infection at age two and died in January 1976 of a generalised chicken pox infection. (An infection is generalised when it is not localised to one particular organ or system.) As with the sailor, retrospective serological testing in the mid 1980s showed both mother and child to be HIV-positive. Most likely the child was infected perinatally by the mother. This sad family history suggests the sailor was infected before 1966 and infected his wife before 1967. If so, HIV was present in Europe by the mid-1960s, if only in this one family the virus had become strong enough to cause AIDS and was transmissible sexually and perinatally. Recently retrospective serological and molecular evidence suggested that HIV-0 infected the Norwegian sailor and his family.

The second sailor is even more mysterious. When he died in 1959, in Manchester, England, a local pathologist performed an autopsy. He found *P. carinii* and cytomegalovirus in the sailor's lungs and herpesvirus in and around his anus. Years later, after AIDS had been recognised, this same pathologist claimed that his patient—now known as the Manchester sailor—was the first reported case.

Studies of frozen tissues from the sailor, preserved by the pathologist, were conducted by virologists in the United Kingdom. They reported finding HIV, but their results could not be replicated in other studies, notably those conducted by the laboratory of David Ho at the Aaron Diamond AIDS Research Center in New York. Using primers able to trace current varieties of HIV, the Ho group showed that the UK studies were most likely contaminated by material from a victim of the current AIDS epidemic.

In a letter to Nature, He reported "serious doubts about the authenticity of the 1959 Manchester man as the first documented case of AIDS due to HIV-I infection." Indeed, Ho's analysis showed that the Manchester man was infected by a strain of virus genetically dissimilar to HIV-1. If the Norway sailor and his family were infected by true HIV in the mid- 1960s, then the virus had changed considerably since it had infected the Manchester sailor in the late 1950s. The Norwegian sailor and his family seem to have suffered from AIDS as we know it, whereas the Manchester man had an early or incomplete form of the disease. This man became seriously ill at age twenty-five in December 1958. He was single and his sexual orientation is unknown. In 1957, with the Royal Navy, he had sailed to Gibraltar and visited Tangier, in Morocco, which even now has very little HIV or AIDS. That was his only trip beyond the United Kingdom. He rapidly developed shortness of breath, nocturnal sweats, weight loss, fatigue and fever.

Early in 1959, deep and painful ulcerations appeared around his mouth and anus. His physicians also noted "scaly brownish lesions on the skin of his back and shoulders." All these problems worsened despite antibiotic therapy, but hormone treatment temporarily improved his appetite and reduced his fever. In the last month of his life, more infections and ulcers appeared on his fingers, lower lip and tongue. He died after a progressive illness of less than two years. At death his emaciated body was entirely covered with small skin lesions. At autopsy, cause of death was revealed to be PCP combined with generalised cytomegalovirus (CMV) infection. Like *P. carinii*, CMV is ubiquitous and rarely harmful to humans except when immunodeficiency allows opportunistic infection. By 1962, thirty-three adult cases of PCP had been reported in the medical literature.

In all but one, the disease was fatal. In almost all cases this pneumonia occurred simultaneously with other infections or tumours. The most commonly described infections were generalised CMV, tuberculosis and cryptococcosis. The tumours were usually leukemias and lymphomas. This picture surely resembles AIDS, but in those days an immunodeficiency could not yet be diagnosed by laboratory means. Many authors who described these cases in the 1950s and 1960s suspected that some underlying cause made the patients fatally vulnerable to infections that normally are innocent. Scientists of the time thought that such lowered resistance was caused either by prolonged hormone therapies or by underlying malignancy. At the same time, they saw that fatal cases of *P. carinii* infection had occurred without any apparent predisposing condition.

Of the thirty-three cases, twenty-seven (82 per cent). were men. About half were in their thirties or forties when they died. All cases seemed sporadic in nature. They were noted mainly in Europe (a few in other continents), but no one suspected that an epidemic was building among young adult males. However, the Norwegian sailor and his family—the only individuals to be confirmed HIV-positive—suggest that HIV was already circulating in the 1960s or even the 1950s. If it killed virtually all of its victims (thirty-two of thirty-three), it had already acquired the ability to cause immunodeficiency with fatal outcome.

If most victims were young single males, this HIV may well have been an early variant of HIV-1 subtype B, the virus that started and still dominates the Western epidemic. HIV-1 B is now known to spread through homosexual (*i.e.*, anal) intercourse more easily than any other HIV type or subtype. HIV-1B is particularly adapted to invade a host through cells in the mucous membrane lining of the anus. If it was the main culprit in those thirty-three early cases, it had already evolved this affinity for the anal mucosa. The evidence seems strong that HIV-1 was among us, waiting only for the opportunity—supplied by the gay emancipation movement of the late 1960s and 1970s—to emerge as the epidemic we know today. The medical literature reveals that, while waiting, it caused small and well-documented epidemics of PCP accompanied by generalised CMV infection in several parts of Europe.

As far as we know, the largest epidemic, which struck very young children, emerged just before World War II and lasted about twenty years. It affected only children in their first year of life, only in continental Europe, but thousands of children died.

The first cases were reported in 1939 from the Baltic port city of Danzig, then in Germany (now Gdansk, in Poland). The epidemic then spread to Switzerland in 1941, to Austria in 1942 and to Italy in 1946, primarily to the east and north of the peninsula. By the end of the 1940s, it had reached Finland, Denmark and Sweden. In Germany itself, the epidemic intensified in the early 1950s. However, although it spread to all corners of the country, it was always most concentrated in the eastern part.

Especially in cities like Leipzig, Dresden and Jena, the fatal cases of PCP reached astonishing numbers. After the 1950s, PCP was increasingly seen in Czechoslovakia and Hungary. In Czechoslovakia alone, five hundred children died of this pneumonia during a five-year period. By the end of the decade, the epidemic had apparently levelled off and, by the early 1960s, it had ceased. How did this epidemic occur and spread? If its basis was an underlying immunodeficiency caused by an HIV-like virus, why did the parents of affected children show no signs of illness? Why did the young victims succumb to acute infection rather than the chronic infection seen today in AIDS patients?

The whole epidemic was confined to a single unit—the so-called Swedish barrack—of the Kweekschool voor Vroedvrouwen, a training hospital for midwives. After 1948, any newborn born too early or with problems was nursed and treated in the Swedish barrack. Separated from their mothers, such newborns normally stayed in the barrack until they reached a weight of 3,000 grams. The unit accommodated forty to forty-four newborns in seventeen small rooms that had beds for two to four patients.

The population of Limburg was unusual because its coal mines drew miners and their families from beyond the Netherlands, in particular from southeastern and eastern Europe. At the training school for midwives, a high percentage of newborns had been fathered by the foreign miners. Their mothers were often unwed local women, who apparently felt more at ease with the midwives than with medical staff at the local hospital.

The PCP epidemic touched only the midwifery school and not the unit for newborns at nearby St. Joseph's Hospital, even though school and hospital shared the same nurses and pediatricians. Several babies born at the school were transferred to St. Joseph's while very sick with PCP, but they did not start a new chain of infections at the hospital. Two babies who were born at St. Joseph's died of PCP. They had never been in the barrack but had occupied beds next to transfers from the barrack who seemed healthy when they arrived. One of these transfers later developed PCP and died, strengthening the case against the barrack as the origin of infection. A serious search by local general practitioners, hospital physicians and pathologists found no other local pockets of infection. The epidemic was apparently confined to a single unit in a single hospital in a single Dutch city. Analysis of all eighty-one PCP cases revealed that the children showed the first signs of disease at minimally about fifty days and maximally one hundred days after birth. The established incubation time for PCP is about one month. Virtually all of us acquire *R. carinii* during our early years, without harm, regardless of our maturity at birth.

These facts strongly suggest that in the Limburg epidemic, some cause of diminished immunity was acquired at or soon after birth. This opened the door to *P. carinii* and CMV. Like *P. carinii,* CMV usually infects us without harm unless it is acquired too early in life. If acquired perinatally, it can cause disease even if immunity is not impaired. When acquired so early, it is usually congenital: it is caught from mothers who carry *P. carinii* and CMV. But normal newborns rarely catch these organisms. Their immune systems protect them until they are old enough to be unharmed by this colonisation. The mothers of newborns in this epidemic showed no manifestations of pneumonia. They did not acquire the cause of immunodeficiency that affected their newborns. The mothers undoubtedly conveyed *R. carinii* and CMV, but what caused immunodeficiency in the newborns? Why did these usually harmless organisms become so deadly? For clues, we must look more closely at the course of the epidemic and its virulence.

First of all, premature birth did not seem to cause the immunodeficiency. During the epidemic, 20 per cent of children born prematurely developed PCP, while 15 per cent of those born at maturity developed the disease. The five-point difference in percentile cannot be considered meaningful, especially since virtually no cases of PCP were observed in the ward for premature newborns at St. Joseph's Hospital. Besides PCP, the children often had CMV complications. In the laboratory, the most striking observation was a hypergammaglobulinemia. This means an abnormally high level of general antibodies—a sign of chronic infectious disease and a hallmark of AIDS in children.

In 1955, the first year of the epidemic, among 230 admissions to the Swedish barrack there were fourteen cases of PCP and/or CMV: an incidence of 6 per cent. Of these first fourteen cases, four died: a mortality rate of 29 percent. The following year, 1956, saw only 6 cases of disease among almost as many admissions—a drop to 3 per cent—and no fatalities. One would assume that the epidemic was over, but the next two years proved otherwise. In 1957, twenty-eight cases of disease occurred among 194 newborns treated in the barrack, raising the incidence to 14 percent. Simultaneously, the death rate rose to 32 per cent of affected infants. So the disease had become not only more frequent but more aggressive.

In 1958, up to August 1, admissions were only fifty-nine because both parents and doctors began to avoid the deadly barrack. Of these, thirty-three newborns developed disease, a majority of those admitted (56 per cent). But while incidence rose, virulence did not change: eleven of the diseased children died, a mortality rate of 33 per cent. In April 1958 after three deaths occurred in rapid succession, it was decided to halt new admissions to the barrack. In July 1958 the last newborns left and immediately thereafter the Swedish barrack was closed forever. No new cases of newborn PCP have occurred in the area since that time.

The highly unusual fatality of the infection strongly points to a preexisting immunodeficiency, that is, a deficiency not caused by premature birth or treatments related to birth. What, then, was special about these children? The only special and consistent factor was their presence in the Swedish barrack. What happened there that did not happen anywhere else? Injections are said to have been given rarely, but blood transfusions are documented in some children, as well as nikethamide injections to improve breathing and sometimes antibiotics.

Protocols and practice for these treatment interventions must have been largely the same at the midwifery school and St. Joseph's Hospital, since the same staff were involved. But how else can we explain the epidemic except to imagine transmission of immunodeficiency by some contaminated intervention? We have seen this happen more than once in the current AIDS epidemic and in various pediatric epidemics. In the 1980s, small but dramatic epidemics of AIDS occurred among children in several hospitals, orphanages and childrens' homes of Eastern Europe. They occurred because reusable syringes and needles were not sterilised between injections and single-use needles and syringes were beyond the budget. In these cases, HIV was spread because the blood of an infected child remained in a syringe that was used to treat an uninfected child.

Another scenario was seen in the Hospital of Leiden University in the Netherlands in 1981. As was customary in those days, premature children receiving intravenous nutrition also received transfusions of plasma. Eleven such children were subsequently found to be infected with HIV and after ten years of follow-up, eight of them had died. Retrospective analysis revealed that all eleven had received plasma from one individual: a homosexual man who donated blood when he was HIV-positive but had no symptoms.

Either of these two scenarios could have brought HIV to the Limburg newborns. It is difficult to explain why such epidemics occurred in widely separated hospitals of Eastern and Western Europe, with different staff and protocols, but did not occur in St. Joseph's Hospital and the nearby Swedish barrack, with their shared staff and protocols. Still, it is easy to imagine how the virus (if HIV played a role) was carried from Eastern Europe to the Netherlands. Most likely, at least one adult—probably a coal miner from Poland, Czechoslovakia, or Italy—brought the virus to Limburg. This one adult could have died from AIDS with little notice.

Like the Norwegian sailor, he could have transmitted the virus to his wife and offspring. His infected wife (or girlfriend) could have given birth in the Swedish barrack to a child who was HIV-positive but seemingly healthy. Unsterilised needles and syringes could have spread the virus from child to child. The less likely scenario, analogous to the Leiden incident, is that a coal miner's HIV-infected blood was used for plasma therapy of newborns. However, no such practice is documented.

The early presence of HIV in Europe seems clear from the sporadic cases of opportunistic infections and tumours, the few cases confirmed HIV-positive (the Norwegian sailor and family) and the epidemics among newborns. These early incarnations of HIV had caused AIDS, but in a strange way. In adults, the 1950s disease looked much like AIDS as we know it today. However, in children the 1950s disease was importantly different from paediatric AIDS as seen since the 1980s. In the earlier time, children sometimes died rapidly after birth—but often they lived and appeared to have cleared the virus. Regarding the Limburg cases, we have no reports of recurrence or delayed effect. No children who recovered from early PCP (with or without CMV) died years later of other manifestations of immunodeficiency. No children who escaped PCP, despite barracks exposure, later showed any sign of immunodeficiency.

Therefore, if the agent of those early epidemics was a variant of HIV-1B, one must assume that its biological characteristics have changed in the intervening thirty to forty years. That a virus of the HIV family may once have caused acute and often fatal disease from which total recovery was possible is not as unlikely as it sounds.

We must then seriously question the widespread notion that today's HIV-1B epidemic arose in the United States, without warning, in the 1980s. It now seems that this Western HIV arose in Europe, with several unheeded warnings, as early as 1939. Certainly some form of the agent was causing sporadic cases in Europe—plus at least one small epidemic among newborns—before launching the major epidemic now seen in Europe and the United States.

In the 1960s and 1970s, probably due to increased opportunity for passage and circulation, the virus apparently changed from a Jembrana-like human virus to the more lethal HIV we know. It changed from a virus from which recovery is possible to one from which recovery is virtually never possible. This change may not have required much time.

SELECTED READINGS

Gagnon, J. H. 1977. *Human Sexualities.* Glenview, IL: Scott Foresman.

Mann, J. M., D.J.M. Tarantola, and T. W. Netter, eds. 1992. *AIDS in the World.* Cambridge: Harvard University Press.

Parker R. G. 1992. Sexual Diversity, Cultural Analysis, and AIDS Education in Brazil. In: *The Time of AIDS: Social Analysis, Theory and Method,* edited by G. Herdt and S. Lindenbaum. Newbury Park, CA: Sage Publications.

Turner, C. F., H. G. Miller, and L. E. Moses. 1989. *AIDS, Sexual Behaviour and Intravenous Drug Use.* Washington, DC: National Academy Press.

7

AIDS Counselling

AIDS is both familiar and mysterious to many mental health professionals. Counsellors and therapists tend to doubt their ability to provide services to HIV-positive clients. Because there is no formal specialisation in the psychological treatment of people with HIV infection, mental health professionals have little training and few sources of consultation in HIV-related issues. Several characteristics of HIV disease should be considered when psychologically assessing HIV-positive clients. The overlap among illness symptoms, medication side effects and vegetative symptoms of psychological distress have been well recognised and tests of depression have been developed for specific use with medical patients and for the elderly.

Overlapping HIV symptoms and psychological distress pose particular problems when assessing depression and anxiety. Overlap occurs for problems in concentration and decision making, negative changes in physical appearance, increased difficulty in social and occupational functioning, sleep disturbances, fatigue, loss of appetite and excessive weight loss.

Additional items reflect worries about physical health and physical attractiveness, declining sexual interests and excessive guilt, all of which may be a part of HIV infection. Similarly, the DSM-IV diagnostic criteria for major depression rely heavily on vegetative symptoms. For a diagnosis with major depression, a person must exhibit five of nine symptoms, five of which overlap with symptoms of HIV disease: significant weight loss, insomnia, fatigue, diminished ability to think or concentrate and psychomotor retardation. Diagnostic criteria for dysthymia reflect similar overlapping physical symptoms.

People with HIV infection who scored above the clinical cutoff on the Beck Depression Inventory reported significantly more HIV symptoms than did nondepressed people, although depressed and non-depressed did not differ in their number of AIDS-defining conditions or T-helper cell counts.

Neurovegetative signs of depression that overlap with HIV symptomatology are particularly important in clinical assessment because sleep disturbances and loss of appetite are among the most common symptoms of depression among people with HIV infection. Hintz et al. also found that HIV-positive individuals have greater sleep disturbance and appetite suppression than members of a depressed HIV-negative comparison group. Although potentially attributable to depression, physical symptoms cannot therefore be used as strong diagnostic indicators of depression without ruling out symptoms of HIV infection.

Similar problems exist in the assessment of anxiety. The Trait Anxiety Inventory, for example, includes two items that reflect fatigue and cognitive confusion. In addition, the Hamilton Rating Scale for Anxiety reflects autonomic reactivity, including gastrointestinal distress and fatigue, symptoms that may also be indicative of progressing HIV infection. Table 1 summarises HIV symptoms that overlap with symptoms of depression and anxiety commonly included in assessment instruments.

Assessment can be made more specific to psychological distress by decomposing assessment instruments into cognitive, affective, behavioural and somatic domains. For example, Kertzner et al. modified the Hamilton Rating Scale for Anxiety in a study of HIV-positive people by omitting items pertaining to somatic distress. Unfortunately, alterations in standardised instruments limit their potential clinical usefulness because norms are rendered invalid and scores from idiosyncratically derived item subsets have unknown psychometric properties.

Table 1
Overlapping symptoms of depression and anxiety with HIV infection

Distress symptom	*HIV-related symptom*
Fatigue/lethargy	Fatigue
Suppressed appetite	Weight loss
Muscle aches	Muscle aches
Insomnia,	
Increased sweating	Night sweats
Gastrointestinal distress	Diarrhoea
Headaches/dizziness,	
Memory lapses	Neurological disturbances

An alternative strategy is to conduct a content analysis of scales. After scoring a scale according to standardized procedures and using available normative data, the scale can be inspected on an item-level basis to see how much scale elevation is accounted for by item subsets. This is a practice that many clinicians routinely use with psychometric tests and that becomes essential in the evaluation of clients with HIV infection. The following example illustrates the importance of item-level analyses by focusing on the symptom comorbidity of the Beck Depression Inventory.

Taken from a study of HIV-positive men and women, a participant scored 18 on the Beck Depression Inventory, where the clinical cutoff for depression is 15. As shown in Table 2, responses from this case indicate that 11 of the 18 points were accounted for by symptoms of depression that overlap with symptoms of HIV infection. Thus, an elevated depression score for this person was partially accounted for by physical and behavioural symptoms of depression that overlap with HIV infection. However, these physical symptoms did not, of course, occur in isolation of cognitive and affective symptoms of depression. On a separate index of HIV-related symptoms and illnesses, this same person indicated that he had persistent fatigue for at least 2 weeks, unintentionally lost at least 10 pounds, had diarrhoea for at least 2 weeks and had muscle aches and cramps. In addition, he had also been diagnosed with two AIDS-defining conditions, lymphoma and HIV wasting syndrome.

Clinical assessment of clients with HIV infection can reduce the potential problems of disease-distress symptom overlap by using tests that do not include physical symptoms as a benchmark for depression and anxiety. Another strategy is to assess clinical constructs that are closely associated with depression and anxiety but do not reflect physical symptomatology.

For example, the Beck Hopelessness Scale correlates with measures of depression, predicts suicidal intentions and does not include physical symptoms. Similarly, assessments of loneliness, guilt and anger provide valuable information concerning negative affective states without reliance on concurrent HIV-related symptomatology. Corollary assessments may be used in combination with depression and anxiety inventories to support or call into question other test results.

Other psychological reactions to HIV infection require similar considerations in clinical assessment. Suicide risk fluctuates during HIV infection and motivations to attempt suicide differ over the course of the disease. Hopelessness and despair are the most likely impetus for attempting suicide early in the course of HIV and exerting personal control and avoiding pain may emerge as reasons for suicide later in infection. Periodic assessments of suicidal ideation, as well other dimensions of psychological distress, are therefore important in the clinical assessment of HIV-positive clients.

When evaluating psychological adaptation to HIV infection, it is essential to not misattribute illness symptoms to distress reactions. Any symptoms of advancing HIV infection require medical evaluation and should not be dismissed as hypochondriasis, somatisation, anxiety, or depression. Another problem in clinical assessment involves evaluating scores against existing norms. Populations most affected by HIV have been the most under-represented in normative samples.

Culture and gender differences in symptom expression and subpopulation base rates may account for some observed distress. These issues underscore the importance of collecting convergent and divergent assessment data when evaluating clients with HIV infection and they suggest that evaluations should be conducted with medical consultation. Caution is needed when screening for depression or anxiety on the basis of most standardised inventories because of the potential for false positives.

Table 2

Item responses on the beck depression inventory by a person with Advanced HIV infection

Beck depression inventory item	*Scorable points*
I feel sad	1
I feel discouraged about the future	1
I do not feel like a failure	0
I don't enjoy things the way I used to	1
I don't feel particularly guilty	0
I don't feel I am being punished	0
I am disappointed in myself	1
I don't feel I am any worse than anybody else	0
I don't have any thought of killing myself	0
I don't cry any more than usual	0
I get annoyed or irritated more easily than I used to	1
I am less interested in other people than I used to be	1
I make decisions about as well as I ever could	0
I am worried that I am looking old or unattractive	1
I have to push myself very hard to do anything	2
I don't sleep as well as I used to	1
I get tired from doing almost nothing	2
My appetite is not as good as it used to be	1
I have lost more than 10 pounds	2
I am worried about physical problems such as aches and pains, upset stomach, or constipation	1
I am less interested in sex than I used to be	1

Assessment of HIV-positive clients almost necessarily demands integrative, multidimensional approaches. Biopsycho-social models are useful in conceptualising evaluations of clients with HIV infection because of their emphasis on behaviour as a function of the nervous system and various other organ systems that, in turn, reflect the functions of tissues, cells and their components.

Each biological and psychological system is interrelated to the others, so that experiences are tied to physiological processes and bodily systems are reciprocally affected by behaviour. In psychological assessment it is therefore essential to inquire about health status, physical symptoms of illness and, perhaps most important, what a person believes about his or her diagnosis and prognosis.

HIV-RELATED PSYCHOTHERAPY

Although the literature on psychotherapy with HIV-positive clients is sparse, available evidence suggests that psychological treatment for clients with HIV infection can be beneficial.

Markowitz *et al.* focused on encouraging and supporting clients to take actions that included the following: becoming involved in their medical care, preventing HIV transmission, tailoring work and social activities to changes in physical functioning and complying with medical treatment recommendations. Therapy also emphasized the here-and-now and framed illness as an opportunity to examine relationships and other issues of importance. Markowitz et al. emphasized exploring options and reinforcing hope. The results of evaluations taken over the course of therapy found that clients showed declines in depressed mood and other signs of emotional distress. Although the study was not a randomised, controlled treatment trial, it does provide data that encourage the use of individual psychotherapy with HIV-positive clients.

There is also evidence that clients with HIV infection and AIDS can benefit from group psychotherapy. Group therapy, however, should not be confused with support groups. By definition, therapy is conducted by trained therapists rather than peer facilitators and therapeutic techniques are a part of the group experience.

Group therapy does encompass similar features of traditional support groups, including disseminating information and fostering supportive relationships, but it goes beyond group experiences through therapeutic interventions. HIV-related group therapy can be based on models designed for other chronic illnesses. S. H. Levine et al. described a psychotherapy group that treated six clients with symptomatic HIV infection. The primary focus of the group was supportive psychotherapy, but it included giving accurate HIV-related information, instruction in adaptive coping strategies and working through losses and anticipatory grief.

The treatment was centered around a supportive atmosphere that reduced HIV-related fears, addressed relationship issues built social supports and found that clients experienced reductions in psychological distress. Most of the current literature on therapy for HIV-positive clients relies upon a cognitive-behavioural therapy orientation.

Cognitive-behavioural approaches

Cognitive behaviour therapy provides several techniques that have been successful in helping clients adjust to other chronic illnesses. Stress management, cognitive restructuring and behavioural self-management skills have been the basis for most interventions with HIV positive clients. For example, Coates et al. described a group intervention that consisted of eight 2-hour weekly sessions and emphasized instruction in systematic relaxation, health habit change such as smoking and alcohol reduction, increasing rest and exercise and stress-management skills. Coates et al. found that participants benefited from participating in the group. Similar cognitive-behavioural group therapies with HIV-positive clients have been effective in reducing psychological distress and enhancing quality of life.

Two well-controlled clinical trials support the value of cognitive-behavioural techniques with HIV-positive clients. One study enrolled gay men into a cognitive-behavioural therapy intervention prior to notification of their HIV antibody test results. Antoni, Baggett, *et al.*, based their treatment on cognitive-behavioural therapy that included the following: behavioural stress management, relaxation skills training, self-monitoring of environmental stressors, stress reappraisal, active coping, enhancing self-efficacy and expanding social networks.

This multicomponent intervention produced significant reductions in psychological distress among men who subsequently tested HIV positive. Antoni et al. concluded that therapy buffered post-HIV-test-notification depression and increased a sense of personal control among men who tested HIV positive.

Relaxation and stress reduction

Standard relaxation exercises have been effective in reducing stress among HIV-positive clients. Alternatively, guided imagery relaxation techniques can be used and may be preferable for clients with medical ailments. If imagery is used in relaxation training, however, it is important that clients do not confuse it with spiritual or alternative healing imagery. Like all behavioural skills training, relaxation requires a thorough assessment, homework, self-monitoring, practice and feedback.

Cognitive restructuring

Refraining and reappraising stressful life events can reduce distress and increase a sense of control. Techniques for cognitive restructuring are described by proponents of self-instruction training. In general, cognitive restructuring involves identifying maladaptive thoughts or self-statements, therapist modelling of adaptive behaviour and messages that guide adaptive behaviours. Cognitive restructuring can effectively reappraise current health status, reframe illness symptoms and maintain a realistic outlook.

Communication skills building

Barriers to self-disclosing HIV infection can be addressed through assertiveness and social skills training and through behavioural problem-solving techniques. Issues of potential rejection and fear of isolation may be addressed using approaches outlined by cognitive-behavioural problem-solving instruction techniques. When self-disclosure of HIV status is desirable or necessary, clients can role-play disclosure in therapy and problem solve potential outcomes. Modelling, practice and corrective feedback can increase client self- efficacy to self-disclose.

Health-related life-style changes

HIV-positive clients often require assistance to change health-related behaviours, including reducing practices that have adverse health effects (*e.g.*, poor nutrition, tobacco use, alcohol and drug use, *etc.*), increasing behaviours that enhance fitness (*e.g.*, rest, exercise, medication compliance, *etc.*) and eliminating sexual and drug-use behaviours that risk HIV transmission. Changes in life-style are broader than narrow behaviour changes and include clusters of behaviours. Step-by-step planning in psychotherapy can set realistic goals. Clients benefit from encouragement and support, as well as from dissolving barriers that prohibit implementing changes. Self-monitoring progress, such as through the use of journals or diaries, is also helpful.

THEMES IN PSYCHOTHERAPY

HIV-positive clients represent a highly diverse population with a wide array of mental health challenges. Clients may seek services for the emotional turmoil of facing HIV and AIDS, to deal with loneliness and isolation or to cope with fears of illness and death. Counsellors and therapists are called upon by HIV-positive clients for accurate information, clarification of medical treatment decisions, spiritual issues, financial concerns and other immediate needs.

HIV-related information and education

Although mental health professionals cannot provide detailed biomedical information or advice to clients, counsellors and therapists can disseminate psychological information and can serve as a valuable information resource. Therapists need a basic understanding of HIV disease to recognise misinformation when it is communicated by clients. Numerous hotlines are readily available and can assist therapists in answering questions and clarifying concerns raised by their HIV-positive clients.

Physicians and public health officials can also serve as consultants. Mental health professionals may educate their clients about psychological issues related to HIV infection and psychological reactions to medical symptomatology. For example, educating clients about the overlap among symptoms of depression, HIV infection and medication side effects can help lead to better understanding and improved psychological adjustment.

- Information and education
- Health promotion
- Disclosing HIV positive status
- Relationships
- Suicide/Hastened death
- Fear of cognitive decline
- Medical treatment issues
- Substance abuse
- Life planning
- Self-esteem and self-worth
- Spirituality
- Redefining quality of life
- Meaningful use of time
- Becoming attached and letting go

Behaviour changes

Altering health-compromising habits and adopting health-promoting behaviours can both improve overall fitness and enhance a sense of personal control. Psychotherapy can help clients alter behaviours with potentially detrimental health effects.

Health psychology offers a rich literature to guide treatments for sleep disorders, nutritional and dietary changes, weight maintenance, medication compliance and other problems that commonly occur in HIV infection. The benefits of health-behaviour change are many, but it is important that clients are not misled to believe that such changes reverse the course of HIV infection. However, changes in health behaviour cannot worsen HIV infection and can improve general health and fitness, clients should be encouraged to make such changes with realistic expectations.

Disclosing HIV seropositivity can be among the greatest challenges facing some HIV-positive clients. Disclosure can result in social sanctions but is necessary to gain certain types of support and to inform sexual and injection drug use partners, dentists and others. In some cases, a therapist may be the only person that a client has told about their HIV status. Disclosure of HIV status can be approached with clients on a person-by-person, case-by-case basis.

Clients may weigh the potential costs and benefits of disclosing their HIV status and evaluate their options for how and when to disclose. Role-playing and rehearsal can occur in therapy, where the therapist helps trouble-shoot potential responses to the disclosure. When clients are unable to bring themselves to disclose to sexual and injecting partners, therapy can offer a vehicle for disclosure by way of couples sessions. Therapists then know that the partner has been told and can provide support to both the client and their partner.

Interpersonal relationships

Family conflicts often predate HIV infection and can become exacerbated after testing HIV positive. Fears and stigmas add to the isolation of HIV-positive clients. Long-term partnered relationships are also disrupted by HIV infection and clients with HIV infection are often kept away from children. Issues of disclosing to partners, maintaining safer sexual relations, fears of future illness and anticipatory loss can weaken relationship bonds. Therapy may therefore involve working through relationship issues and, when appropriate, include partners or family members.

Recurrent suicide risk

The risk for suicide among HIV-positive clients occurs within two distinct contexts. Suicidal ideations can occur in conjunction with hopelessness and clinical depression.

Alternatively, clients may view suicide as a reasonable option in HIV infection. Thus, suicide interventions depend on the meaning of suicidal ideations and the motivation behind suicide intentions.

Monitoring suicide risk is a continuous process. HIV-positive clients are reminded of their mortality by the deaths of others, the onset of symptoms, anniversaries of HIV testing and the deaths of friends. Therapists must have clear values on hastened death and partner-assisted hastened death so that they can remain non-judgemental when dealing with these serious issues in therapy.

Neuropsychological effects of HIV infection

Perceptions of cognitive changes in relation to HIV infection require regular re-evaluation. Mental status can be monitored and client attributions of changes should be assessed. Because many do not experience neuropsychological impairment even late in the course of AIDS, clients can be reassured that cognitive limitations are not necessarily inevitable. If neuropsychological symptoms are confirmed by a neuropsychological consultant, therapists can assist clients in adapting to cognitive decline or vision impairment. Clients should be encouraged to be patient with themselves because completing complex tasks may require more time.

Counselling HIV-positive clients

Mental health services occur within a broad spectrum of care for most HIV-positive clients. Communication among providers is therefore necessary because treatment components can be interactive. For example, antiretroviral drugs have behaviour-related side effects such as fatigue and peripheral neuropathy and certain antidepressant and cognitive performance-enhancing medications may interact with treatments of HIV infection. Permission to release and obtain information from other professionals involved in the care of HIV-positive clients should be routine. Multidisciplinary inpatient treatment teams can be emulated for outpatients by opening communication lines and building a network of cooperative relationships.

Psychotherapy can also help clients address medically related concerns, including treatment attitudes, compliance and life-and-death issues. Mental health professionals can support clients who have selected a course of treatment and have been compliant. Clinicians can also help their HIV-positive clients clarify their wishes for terminal care, such as life support options and resuscitation.

Therapy can help clarify such issues for clients and sessions can be used to problem solve barriers and role-play communicating desires for terminal care with physicians. Terminal care should be discussed early in the course of HIV infection to avoid later cognitive decline that will increase the difficulty of decision making.

Substance abuse treatment

Clients with injection drug using histories can be particularly difficult to treat because of the strong addictive qualities of injected drugs and issues related to potential transmission of HIV to needle-sharing partners. All types of substance use, including alcohol, can serve as avoidance coping strategies and can raise the risk for engaging in HIV-transmitting behaviours. Psychotherapy can assist HIV-positive clients who should be motivated to stop using substances by helping them replace drug use with adaptive coping behaviours. However, specialised treatment may be necessary for substance abusive clients.

Planning for the future

HIV-positive clients become acutely aware of mortality and recognise that their time is limited. Goals for therapy therefore require attention to both short-term and long-term time lines. Clients should be encouraged to establish priorities for therapy and to identify a primary goal. Working with a therapist, clients can translate their primary goal into smaller, short-term goals. HIV-positive clients are often inclined to emphasize the near future and to cut short lifelong aspirations. A sense of realistic optimism, however, can allow clients to restore long-term goals, again stated in terms of concrete steps.

Self-esteem and self-worth

Working through life issues and moving toward achieving goals is a self-enhancing process. Because clients with a life-threatening illness may have special needs to enhance their self-esteem, therapy can work toward achieving greater self-acceptance. One therapeutic technique that is useful in this regard is life review, where clients are guided through a self-examination of life transitions. People with chronic illnesses commonly think about their past to gain a sense of closure. Therapy can therefore provide structure and support a life review process.

Spirituality

Clients with HIV infection are often estranged from formal religious institutions and may therefore express unmet spiritual needs. Therapists can help clients clarify their values and identify spiritual needs in the context of psychotherapy. Therapy can also take the form of developing strategies for exploring traditional and non-traditional spiritual practices. Clients may wish to seek guidance from clergy and can use therapy as a means of problem solving barriers and evaluating options to meet their spiritual needs.

Redefining quality of life

Needs and abilities change as a function of HIV infection. Adjustments in therapy goals, focus and course are therefore required as HIV infection progresses. In particular, quality of life must be continuously evaluated and redefined over the course of illness. Pain, health status, physical functioning, social relationships and energy level contribute to the quality of life. When activities are disrupted and abilities are impaired, therapists can help find new activities that match current abilities and reframe quality of life along those lines.

Unemployment, disability and activity restrictions lead to boredom and other forms of discontent. Many HIV-positive clients state that quality use of their time is one of their primary concerns. Counsellors and therapists may help clients evaluate their physical capabilities and work through options to increase life satisfaction. Creativity and productivity can move HIV-positive clients out of passive victim roles. Volunteering to help others, rediscovering hobbies and interests, taking time for oneself and focusing on relationships are examples of ways to enhance a sense of meaning.

Professionals who treat patients suffering from life-threatening illnesses undergo a great deal of stress. Hopelessness, fear of death, spiritual crisis and recognising one's own mortality are common themes in terminal illness. As much as any area of psychotherapy, boundaries between the client and therapist can be blurred by the universality of death and mortality, issues that many therapists themselves have not worked through. A clear sense of one's own views on death and dying will enable clinicians to better serve their HIV-positive clients.

PSYCHOPHARMACOLOGICAL TREATMENTS

An emerging body of research suggests that medications are effective in treating HIV-positive clients and the risk of adverse effects appear minimal. Markowitz, Rabkin and Perry reviewed clinical trials of antidepressant medications in HIV infection and found that three controlled studies of imipramine demonstrated the efficacy of this drug with HIV-positive clients. Similar results were reported with other antidepressants as well as stimulants used to treat depression. The use of antidepressants with HIV-positive clients is supported by the available research. Unfortunately, studies evaluating anti-anxiety and other classes of psychiatric medications are not available.

ISSUES FOR WOMEN

HIV-positive women experience the medical, social and psychological aspects of the HIV disease differently than men. Although HIV appears to take the same course in women as it does in men, immune-compromised women are susceptible to a number of gynaecology infections and cancers that have only recently been recognised.

In addition, because most early studies of the natural history of HIV disease and the majority of treatment studies have only included gay men, less is known about HIV infection and effects of treatment among women. In terms of social aspects of HIV disease, women suffer more prejudices for sexually contracting HIV infection than do men.

Women are also subject to the stress of being a caretaker for an HIV-positive partner. Furthermore, the clinical picture for women is potentially complicated by pregnancy. Many women learn they are HIV positive through prenatal screening, a nearly routine test in most urban hospitals. If testing occurs early in pregnancy, women must decide whether to terminate in light of potential perinatal HIV transmission. Pregnant women must also consider the use of antiretroviral medications that may help protect the fetus against infection but with risk of unknown teratogenic effects. Finally, women who already have children are burdened with assuring their care in anticipation of becoming disabled and ultimately, dying.

Studies of psychological issues facing women with HIV infection have been few. Little information is therefore available to guide the treatment of women with HIV infection. The following case description illustrates several issues facing women with HIV infection. The case description is accurate with respect to all clinically relevant details, with identifiable characteristics altered to protect the client's identity.

> The client was a 23-year-old Mexican American woman diagnosed with HIV infection 3 months earlier through prenatal HIV screening. She was asymptomatic for HIV infection and was 8 months pregnant at the time of referral, but has since given birth. Maria has two children, including her newborn and is engaged to be married. Her fiance, however, tested HIV negative. She presented in therapy with symptoms of depression and anxiety related to her health and the uncertainty of her newborn's HIV status.
>
> Maria expressed great concern regarding potential perinatal transmission of HIV, providing care for her children after her death, disclosing her HIV status to others close to her and issues of communication and support in her family and social relationships. She has disclosed her HIV status to her fiance and best friend, the latter of whom she sees only infrequently. Her

fiance prefers not to discuss HIV-related issues. Maria fears her family's reaction to her HIV status and has not disclosed it to them.

Maria reported the following symptoms of depression: decreased interest in activities, depressed mood, diurnal mood variation, tearfulness, loss of energy, feelings of hopelessness and being overwhelmed, diminished ability to concentrate and recurrent thoughts of death. She denied sleep disturbance, changes in appetite and suicidal ideation. Maria experienced an exacerbation in her depression following the birth of her child and HIV-antibody screening conducted for her older son. Maria therefore met diagnostic criteria for a DSM-IV diagnosis of major depression. Her emotional reaction was related to her recent knowledge of her HIV status, perceived lack of social support and concerns for her future and for her children.

Maria reported a history of depression and alcohol use during her adolescence. She received inpatient psychiatric treatment for depression and truancy. Maria was physically abused by her mother and reported an extensive family history of mental illness. Maria acknowledged previous maladaptive ways of coping and an attempted suicide during her adolescence. She described her previous psychological treatment as successful, through both psychotherapy and antidepressant medication.

The following short-term treatment goals were identified: (a) increasing the amount and quality of social support, including informing family members of HIV status and seeking an HIV-related support group; (b) developing adaptive coping strategies, initially through cognitive and behavioural approaches, to cope with her situation and to alleviate depression; and (c) increasing communication and support related to HIV issues with her partner. Following improved adjustment and adaptive coping, Maria identified a long-term therapy goal of addressing unresolved issues related to the future care of her children as her HIV infection progresses and to the physical abuse and perceived abandonment resulting from her mother's suicide.

> Psychotherapeutic progress included an increase in social support through communication skills development and improved self-esteem, probably because of a supportive therapeutic relationship and successful experiences with assertiveness. Maria subsequently informed two family members of her HIV status and dealt effectively with their emotional reactions, which were initially supportive. Her older child tested negative for HIV antibodies and she is waiting the testing period to confirm her newborn's HIV serostatus. Maria continues to feel anxious and depressed in relation to ongoing caregiving concerns and her children's welfare following her death. She is currently in good health and has received assistance from a community-based organisation in the form of social services. Maria continues to have difficulty in communicating and receiving emotional support from her fiance, as well as maintaining consistent safer sexual behaviours. Couples therapy was considered to deal with her complex relationship issues.

This case, although by no means representative, illustrates several salient issues that arise for women with HIV. The case involved a woman who was pregnant and who had a previous child and weak social supports. The case was also complicated because the client contracted HIV infection outside of her current relationship. Because most research has disproportionately sampled men, particularly white gay men, little is known about the interactions of these complex issues and how they affect therapy.

CONFIDENTIALITY

Privacy is a central element in effective psychotherapy. Therapists, however, are obligated to break confidentiality under certain circumstances. Issues of duty to protect are among the greatest HIV-related ethical and legal concerns among mental health professionals because of the role of confidentiality in professional relationships. Perceptions of dangerousness and identification of third parties who may be at risk have brought issues raised by the widely noted *Thrasoff v. Regents of California.*

For Thrasoff to apply, there must be a foreseeable danger to an identifiable party as a result of a client's planned behaviour. The Thrasoff ruling involves an obligation for professionals to use reasonable care to protect intended victims when danger is reasonably predicted. The relationship between HIV risk and Thrasoff is highlighted by communicable diseases having long been considered a valid reason to break professional confidentiality to prevent the spread of illness. In fact, Thrasoff itself was based on court decisions that ruled that physicians have a duty to act to protect when they know patients with infectious diseases threaten others.

The relationship between HIV risk and Thrasoff is not, however, as clear as it may first seem. Thrasoff is usually associated with a direct verbal threat. However, HIV-positive clients are unlikely to use their infection to harm another person intentionally. Instead, concerns revolve around the failure to take precaution. In addition most people at risk of exposure to HIV are not easy for clinicians to identify. Duty to protect only extends to people who can be identified and who could reasonably be harmed. Unlike in Thrasoff, potential victims of HIV transmission are probably already aware of the risks associated with their own behaviour, given that high-risk practices are well known and everyone is advised to protect themselves.

The American Medical Association recommends that when physicians know that an HIV-positive patient is endangering a third party, they should be persuaded to stop engaging in risk behaviours. If the person fails to comply, the physician should notify public health authorities and if the authorities do not act, the physician should notify the endangered party him or herself.

Similarly, the Canadian Medical Association states that physicians can ethically disclose a patient's HIV status to a spouse when the patient is unwilling to inform him or her. Following these general parameters, the American Psychiatric Association has proposed its own guidelines. A policy statement recommends that psychiatrists work with all patients to reduce their risk for HIV transmission, regardless of serostatus and be competent in counselling about HIV testing. In terms of protecting third parties, the policy statement reads as follows:

> In a situation where a psychiatrist received convincing clinical information that the patient is infected with HIV, the psychiatrist should advise and work with the patient either to obtain agreement to cease behaviour that places others at risk of infection or to notify individuals who may be at continuing risk of exposure. If a patient refuses to agree to change behaviour or to notify the persons at ongoing risk or if the psychiatrist has good reason to believe that the patient has failed to or is unable to comply with this agreement, it is ethically permissible for the psychiatrist to notify identifiable persons who the psychiatrist believes to be in danger of contracting the virus, or to arrange for public health authorities to do so.

The American Psychiatric Association also states that it is ethically permissible to notify public health authorities when a patient's behaviour constitutes a risk to people who cannot be identified, as well as to past sexual or drug-injecting partners. Similar guidelines were established for psychiatric inpatients, as well by other professions, including social workers.

Protective actions can include interventions to stop their client's risk behaviour and therefore eliminate potential harm. When clients are noncompliant, therapists may notify public health authorities of the danger rather than directly warn the third party. Partner notification falls within the professional role of public health workers rather than that of psychotherapists and counsellors. Certain clients, such as those who are sexually impulsive, manic, psychotic, or antisocial, may require involuntary hospitalisation, in effect isolating them from potential victims.

Hospitalisation should, however, only be used to treat mental illness; decisions to quarantine again fall within professional roles of public health authorities, not mental health professionals. Finally, clients should be informed of the limits of confidentiality before they start treatment as a part of routine informed consent procedures. Informing clients that information pertaining to potential harm to others must be reported to appropriate authorities provides clinicians with a stated basis for disclosing otherwise confidential information.

SEXUAL RISK-REDUCTION COUNSELLING

Cessation of all fluid-exchanging sexual and drug-using behaviours is essential among persons with HIV infection to protect others from infection, as well as to protect themselves from reinfection and contracting other sexually transmitted pathogens. Behaviours that confer high risk for HIV transmission are difficult to change because they are highly reinforcing, sustained over long periods of time, driven by biological needs and interwoven with aspects of self-concept, affection and belongingness.

Abstinence from sexual intercourse or consistent practice of safer sex is difficult to achieve and can require support. In many cases, psychotherapy provides an environment for modifying high-risk behavioural practices.

According to the Centers for Disease Control and Prevention, personalised risk-reduction counselling should include accurate information about HIV transmission, addressing personal needs and life circumstances related to risk behaviours; skills to reduce risk effectively; and a realistic, feasible plan of risk reduction. Counselling should also be culturally competent, developmentally appropriate and sensitive to issues, of sexual orientation and gender.

Strategies that have to date demonstrated reductions in high-risk sexual behaviours among HIV-risk populations have been based on principles of social cognitive theory. Components of effective interventions include providing accurate information pertaining to HIV transmission, personal risk sensitisation, identifying and managing behaviour-change barriers, instruction in proper condom use and needle cleaning and training in interpersonal assertiveness and other communication skills necessary to develop and maintain lower-risk relationships. Cognitive-behavioural interventions are known to decrease rates of unprotected sexual intercourse among homosexually active men, inner-city women, chronic mentally ill adults, African American adolescent males and runaway adolescents. In most studies, multi-session group interventions produce substantial reductions in high-risk sexual practices.

Cognitive-behavioural skills training interventions have used principles based on social cognitive theory and cognitive-behavioural skills training techniques, including risk and behaviour-change education, modelling relationship skills related to risk reduction, generating behavioural self-management strategies, providing problem-solving skills for risk-producing situations, emphasizing the importance of practice for effective behaviour change and providing opportunities for guided practice with corrective feedback.

Basic HIV education

HIV-positive clients must possess accurate and up-to-date information about HIV risk behaviours. An evaluation of the client's knowledge of HIV risk transmission factors can be guided by using an objective test of AIDS knowledge. Going over specific knowledge areas in sessions can help clarify information needs. Therapists may consult with local health departments and AIDS service organizations for educational materials. Numerous pamphlets and videotapes are available and can support therapy-based education. Counsellors should be able to clarify misconceptions, dispel myths about AIDS and supply correct information to replace misinformation.

Personal risk assessment

Clients should be guided through a personal assessment of their own behavioural risk histories and identify individual life situations that contribute to risk. A comprehensive sexual history is therefore necessary and should include questions about sexual experimentation, sexual trade, previous sexually transmitted diseases, perceived risk of sexual partners and use of condoms. A useful tool for guiding a client through a personal risk assessment is to have them place their behaviour on a risk continuum, indicating the degree to which their behaviour has placed them at risk. An assessment of the client's readiness to change is also necessary and motivational counselling may be needed before instituting a program for behaviour change.

Condom use and needle-cleaning instructions

Many clients can benefit from instruction in the proper use of condoms and needle cleaning. The greatest obstacles to condom use are attitudes regarding reduced sensation and inconvenience. Clients focus on sensations and total sexual acts to increase sexual satisfaction with condoms can effectively change attitudes. Acknowledging benefits of condoms, such as protection from sexually transmitted diseases and increased duration of penile erection can also help reframe condom attitudes. The proper use of condoms should be instructed using the following steps: (a) carefully opening the package and not damaging the latex, (b) pinching the tip of the condom to assure a reservoir and remove air, (c) rolling the condom from the tip of the head of the penis and of the way back to the base, (d) removing the condom immediately after intercourse and disposing of it after one use.

It is also important to educate clients that latex condoms with water-based, not water-soluble, lubricants protect against infections. Information and instruction in the now-available condom-like barriers for women should also be discussed. The female condom, although more expensive than penile condoms, offers women more control in safer sex decisions.

Clients who use injection drugs should also be instructed in cleaning injection equipment in the following way: (a) prepare a bleach-water solution using one part bleach to nine parts water, (b) syphon in the solution through the needle to fill the syringe, (c) flush all of the solution through the needle, (d) repeat this action twice, (e) rinse in water twice after cleaning. Of course, it is best not to share needles at all. The use of clean needles relies heavily on policy regarding injection equipment availability and needle exchange. Studies show that needle exchange reduces HIV infection rates and people should be encouraged to use sterile needles whenever possible.

Behaviour and self-management skills

Clients can be instructed to identify environmental and cognitive-affective cues that serve as "triggers" for high-risk situations, including mood states, substance use, settings and sexual partner characteristics. Strategies for handling risk-related cues and situations may include avoiding certain partners, places, or substance use in relation to se⁻ual situations.

Another important aspect of behavioural self-management is the use of self-monitoring techniques. Journals, diaries and logs of personal risk behaviour as well as risk behaviour triggers can have reactive effects and reduce risk. Self-monitoring also provides a useful assessment technique and can help identify particularly difficult risk situations, which may then be addressed through problem solving and action planning.

Identification of barriers to risk reduction can be achieved in therapy. Behavioural self-management of barriers can be placed in the context of a problem-solving model in which clients (a) identify personal problem situations, (b) gather information for possible solutions, (c) evaluate options and (d) plan a course of action. Step-by-step plans developed with clients should be realistic and feasible.

Sexual communication skills

Therapy can focus on the role of sexual negotiation, assertiveness and refusal skills to reduce risk for HIV infection. Increasing skills for disclosing HIV serostatus, resisting partner coercion to engage in sexual intercourse without condoms and increasing comfort in discussing safer sex with partners in advance of sexual activity can be accomplished through instruction, role-play modelling, practice in communicating sexual decisions and discussing individual limits to behaviour change. Clients can identify past situations of high risk and generate statements that would have led to a lower risk. Emphasis can be placed on effective communication of feelings and sexual behaviour limits prior to entering sexual situations.

Using communication techniques to reduce risk may have special implications for women because of sexual double standards placed on talking about sex. It is important that efforts by women to protect themselves do not inadvertently result in endangerment. Negotiating safer sex may therefore be placed in the context of health and reproductive needs, reducing the possibility of suspicion and angry reactions to initiating safer sex discussions.

Although these intervention components have been effective in group formats, they can also be instituted in individual therapy. Research continues to identify new and effective strategies for HIV risk reduction that vary for men and women, sexual orientation group; ethnic groups, age groups and types of relationships. As new intervention approaches for HIV prevention emerge, there will be additional procedures available to therapists. Methods of adapting these procedures to psychotherapy are evolving and should become available to clinicians.

HIV infection emerged as a global health threat faster than any previous disease in history. AIDS is the first disease to establish itself as a leading cause of death within the same decade of its discovery and is now the number one cause of death among men and women between the ages of 25 and 44. By 1986 AIDS was responsible for 38 per cent of all deaths among San Francisco men ages 20 to 49 and this figure increased to 61 per cent in 1990. By the end of 1993, 220,871 people had died of an AIDS-related condition in the United States, 73 per cent of whom were been 25 and 44 years old.

In contrast with other causes of death, AIDS has steadily increased each year over the past decade. The clinical course of HIV infection begins at the time of virus exposure and ends at the time of death from AIDS-related illnesses. Because AIDS is a new disease, our knowledge of its mechanisms is still incomplete.

Furthermore, most of what is currently known about HIV disease comes from studies of men who sexually contracted the virus from other men, people living in major urban centers who became infected through injection drug use and individuals with blood clotting disorders. Most information about the natural progression of HIV disease comes from the Multicenter AIDS Cohort Study (MACS), which enrolled 4,955 homosexual and bisexual men from four cities (Baltimore, Chicago, Los Angeles and Pittsburgh) and followed them at 6-month assessment intervals. The objective was to identify and study gay men who were HIV seropositive, men who became HIV infected during the study and men who remained seronegative. MACS investigators sought information relevant to developing HIV prevention programs and early treatment strategies. Information from a few similar cohorts supplements results reported from MACS, including the San Francisco City Cohort, San Francisco General Hospital Cohort, the Men's Health Study and the Vancouver Lymphadenopathy-AIDS Study. Because these cohorts comprised gay and bisexual men, the generalisation of results to women and ethnic minorities is highly limited.

HIV infection is silent for most of its duration, only becoming overtly symptomatic at its later stages. The natural history of HIV infection is highly variable and changes over the course of the epidemic. There is now considerable evidence that people infected with HIV will develop AIDS and will die of an AIDS-related illness. The length of time from infection to an AIDS-related condition varies from as short as 1 year to 15 years or longer. Studies have shown that 5 per cent to 10 per cent of HIV-infected people progress to AIDS within 4 years and nearly 50 per cent develop AIDS by 10 years after initial infection.

No single factor or combination of factors accounts for variability in HIV progression. Differences in rates of decline occur among individuals who contract HIV through different modes of transmission.

Most studies have, however, found that the average duration from time of HIV infection to AIDS, in the absence of treatment, is between 7 and 10 years. The time between contracting HIV and developing AIDS is for the most part characterised by an absence of serious illness. Several descriptive systems are available for staging HIV disease. In an early classification scheme, the CDC had a four-stage progressive model that included an acute infection syndrome, a long period of asymptomatic infection, the development of persistent generalised lymphadenopathy (enlarged lymph nodes) and later disease manifestations. A second staging system developed by CDC included an expanded list of diseases associated with AIDS and an early symptomatic phase of disease referred to AIDS-related complex. In the 1987 CDC system as shown in Table 3, stages I and II consist of asymptomatic periods, stage III is characterised by chronic lymphadeno-pathy and the substages of stage IV represent later phases. More recent staging systems rely on tracking the number of T-helper lymphocyte cells over the course of infection.

Table 3

Centers for disease control staging system for human immunodeficiency virus infection

Stage	*Description*
I	Actuate HIV infections; asymptomatic or possible acute viral reaction latent infection
II	Latent infection
III	Chronic lymphadenopathy
IV-A	Constitutional symptoms: weight loss, fever, chronic diarrhoea
IV-B	HIV-induced neuropathology: dementia, myelopathy, peripheral neuropathy
IV-C	Opportunistic infections
IV-D	HIV-associated tumours
IV-E	Other conditions

The course of HIV infection varies across subpopulations. For example, perinatally HIV-infected infants and children have shorter survival times compared with adolescents and adults. Although there are few significant differences between HIV-positive and negative newborns at birth HIV-positive infants become ill early, with a median onset of symptoms between 8 and 10 months of age and the majority of children becoming ill within one year. HIV-positive infants have higher rates of certain complications, such as neurological diseases, which occur in 30 per cent to 60 per cent of infected infants.

Failure to thrive is also common, as are delays in developmental milestones and the actual loss of milestones once achieved. HIV-positive infants are particularly susceptible to disease because HIV inhibits the development of the immature immune system, accelerating the course of HIV infection. The criteria for diagnosing AIDS in infants and children consist of the same AIDS-defining conditions that diagnose AIDS in adults, along with other specific and recurrent infections. Unlike infants and young children, the clinical progression of AIDS for adolescents is more like that for adults. The following sections review HIV disease processes from the point of infection to later phases of illness.

PRIMARY HIV INFECTION

The body mounts an immune reaction that is ineffective in stopping HIV infection, following the introduction of HIV into the bloodstream. In response to HIV, the body may react with a brief period of acute infection symptoms. The usual time that lapses between exposure and acute illness is about two to four weeks, with the duration of symptoms lasting only one to two weeks. Acute retroviral illness, when it does occur, is the earliest clinically recognisable event in the natural history of HIV infection. Response to retroviral infection is similar to vague symptoms of mononucleosis.

However, retroviral infection actually consists of a distinct and recognisable clinical syndrome. Most typically, acute HIV symptom illness, or primary HIV infection, presents with persistent fever, lethargy, malaise, muscle weakness, headache, pain in or around the eyes, sensitivity to bright light, sore throat and skin rashes. In most cases, primary HIV infection symptoms resolve themselves and usually do not recur. Not all people infected with HIV, however, develop symptoms of primary infection. Studies have found that between 40 per cent and 90 per cent of individuals experience an acute response to HIV infection. Symptoms occur among people infected through each major route of HIV transmission and, at present, there is no conclusive evidence that any particular group is more likely to develop symptomatic acute illness. In addition to the aforementioned early symptoms, HIV-positive persons may develop persistent generalised lymphadenopathy, defined by enlarged lymph nodes that are detectable by touch and remain enlarged for a minimum of three months.

Swollen lymph nodes in the armpits, neck, or groin are common in HIV infection, as well as in other viral infections, with 70 per cent of HIV-positive persons having swollen nodes within the first few weeks of infection. In the case of HIV infection, swollen lymph nodes are the result of disseminated HIV throughout the lymphatic system. Most studies show that persistent lymphadenopathy does not have prognostic value for disease progression towards AIDS. Following acute symptoms of HIV infection, although not dependent on the occurrence of such symptoms, antibodies are produced against HIV.

Establishing HIV antibodies, or seroconversion to HIV, most likely results after a threshold of HIV replication has occurred and depends on the immune competency of the host to mount the antibody response. On average, HIV antibodies are detectable through serological testing slightly more than 2 months after viral transmission and 95 per cent of HIV-infected individuals develop antibodies within 6 months of becoming infected.

However, the incubation period for HIV may last longer than 6 months and in rare cases incubation may last 2 to 3 years. Variability in establishing HIV antibodies can come from numerous factors, including the virulence of viral strains, the dose of virus transmitted, the frequency of exposure and an individual's immune response. Once antibodies have developed, they are detectable through HIV testing.

HIV TESTING

Some diagnostic tests for HIV infection involve detecting HIV genetic material directly in blood cells or actually culturing the virus. However, the most widely used tests identify antibodies to the virus rather than the presence of HIV itself Antibodies produced by the immune system provide immunologic "footprints" to viral infection. Antibody tests are safer for laboratories to perform than actual viral-detection procedures because antibody tests do not require direct contact with HIV. Antibody tests also tend to be less expensive than viral cultures and genetic testing. The standard procedures for HIV antibody testing involve providing written informed consent, pre-test counselling for 30 to 90 minutes (including an explanation of the test), discussions of limited confidentiality when tests are not anonymous, personalised risk assessments and exploration of individual concerns.

The test procedure itself involves drawing blood and sending samples for laboratory analysis. Post-test result notification and counselling usually occur about two weeks after the initial visit. Blood collected for testing is first subjected to an enzyme-linked immunosorbent assay (ELISA) that tests for antibodies to HIV. ELISA tests are done first because they are highly sensitive to HIV antibodies. If an ELISA test is negative, it is highly improbable that the person is HIV infected. In other words, false negative results from an ELISA test are rare. Positive ELISA tests must be repeated because the procedure is not specific to HIV antibodies. Thus, a greater likelihood exists that an ELISA result will be a false positive. For this reason, ELISA tests are used to screen blood samples for HIV antibodies.

After a blood specimen receives a repeated positive ELISA, the test is confirmed using a western blot procedure. Like ELISA, western blot detects HIV antibodies, but western blot is highly specific because it determines the exact antigens toward which antibodies are directed. A positive western blot result means detection of two out of three precise antigen groups from components of HIV. This level of specificity reduces the chances of false positive results to an extremely low probability. Thus, both a positive repeated ELISA screening test and a positive western blot confirmatory test are required for diagnosis of HIV infection.

HIV antibody testing is now among the most accurate diagnostic tools in medicine. In tests that indicate a false negative result (*i.e.*, that the person is not found infected when he or she really is infected), the most common cause is that the blood sample was collected during the incubation window period before the presence of HIV antibodies.

A person cannot, therefore, know that they are HIV infected during the first month or two of infection, although HIV can be transmitted to others during this time. The potential for false negative tests requires that all persons who receive this result be tested again approximately 3 months later. People who test HIV-positive and have no identifiable risk history should also be retested, although false positive test results only occur because of laboratory errors.

In addition to receiving either a positive or a negative result, a third possible outcome is an, indeterminate result: neither conclusively positive nor negative. Indeterminate HIV test results usually occur when the ELISA test is positive and only one of the two required specific antigens is detected by western blot.

Ambiguous results occur with respect to both HIV-1 and HIV-2 antibody tests and are most commonly found among individuals infected with HIV who are in the process of developing antibodies and require that the test be repeated 2 to 6 months later. HIV testing is the only reliable means of determining HIV infection. Even after symptoms, many HIV-related illnesses can be caused by non-HIV immune-suppressing conditions. Thus, individuals with symptoms should be tested for HIV antibodies rather than assuming that they are HIV infected on the basis of illness alone.

ASYMPTOMATIC HIV INFECTION

The virus is actively depleting T-helper lymphocytes during clinically asymptomatic phases and HIV is transmittable to others during this time. It was once thought that HIV replicated less during asymptomatic periods, primarily because of low concentrations of virus in the bloodstream. Although termed a latency period, asymptomatic HIV infection does not constitute a time of microbiological inactivity.

Recent studies have shown that HIV is productive in lymph nodes when patients are symptom free. Following years of destruction, the immune system slowly degenerates, increasing vulnerability to illness. The primary target of

HIV, T-helper lymphocytes, is one of three types of thymus-originating cells (T-cells) of the immune system. These cells function to distinguish self from nonself and rid the body of foreign agents. Cytotoxic T-cells identify and destroy infectious agents, suppressor T-cells reduce immune responses and T-helper cells induce responses from several branches of the immune system.

T-helper lymphocytes are the only of the three that express the CD4 surface receptor and HIV therefore binds with and infects these cells. T-helper lymphocytes have several functions, including the induction of non-T-helper cell activity. Cell-mediated immunity results from the production of cytokines that guide a number of immunologic responses. For example, T-helper lymphocytes mediate through cytokines the activity of natural killer cells, which in turn destroy viral-infected and certain cancerous cells. Impaired natural killer-cell activity is an outcome of T-helper cell dysfunction. Cytokines also direct the proliferation and maturation of several other immune cells.

Decreased numbers of T-helper lymphocytes were among the first immunologic abnormalities described in patients with AIDS. Over the course of HIV infection, the average decline in T-helper lymphocytes ranges from 50 to 80 cells/mm^3 per year. At this rate, over a 10-year period, T-helper cell counts drop to between 200 cells/mm^3 and 0 cells/mm^3, increasing vulnerability to infections and malignancies. The single best predictor of developing AIDS in HIV-positive gay men is the rate of T-helper cell decline and blood concentration of T-helpers relative to other immune cells.

Because the number of T-helper cells is inversely related to symptoms, low T-helper cell counts indicate impending illness. During asymptomatic periods, T-helper cell counts are usually between 500 and 200 cells/mm^3, although nearly half of individuals with counts below 200 cells/mm^3 are also asymptomatic at any given time. T-helper cell counts are a marker for HIV disease progression, but they are limited by extreme fluctuations because of a number of factors, including variability in laboratory procedures and changes in cell concentrations over diurnal cycles.

Changes in cell counts are also difficult to interpret because there are no normative data for HIV-infected patients and non-infected risk groups. Despite their limitations, T-helper lymphocyte counts set guidelines for prognostic decisions, for initiating medications that suppress HIV production and for determining when to initiate prophylaxis against opportunistic illnesses. Thus, the risk for AIDS-related conditions increases over the course of HIV infection and the most reliable marker for disease progression is the number of functional T-helper lymphocytes present in the immune system.

Vulnerability to disease increases as the immune system loses T-helper cells and T-helper-cell-mediated immunity. Although immune-system suppression does not necessarily mean symptomatic illness, having an HIV-related illness does suggest severe immune suppression.

Only 2 per cent of cases progress to AIDS within 2 years of becoming infected, whereas as many as 10 per cent progress to AIDS within 4 years. The mean length of time between infection and developing AIDS is 8 to 10 years among homosexually active men and it is considerably shorter for adults who contracted HIV through blood transfusions. Evidence suggests, however, that the interval between infection and illness is lengthening as a result of advances in medical treatments.

The variable clinical manifestations of HIV infection have led to several hypotheses concerning factors that facilitate or inhibit the virus. There are several potential influences on the duration and course of most infectious diseases, including socio-demographic factors, general health status, nutrition, previous illness history, genetic immune factors, variations in viral strains and seasons of the year. Among socio-demographic characteristics, age is consistently associated with HIV progression, with older people having more rapid rates of immune suppression.

Moss and Bacchetti found that people infected with HIV at ages over 40 years were more likely to become ill sooner than individuals infected at younger ages. Men who were infected after age 30 also have poorer survival than their younger-age counterparts. Similarly, once diagnosed with AIDS, older adults die sooner than younger adults.

Ethnic minorities demonstrate a more rapid decline in T-helper lymphocytes than do whites *a*nd there are ethnic differences in the relative frequency of AIDS-related illnesses. Sex differences in prognosis have also been suggested; men live longer after an AIDS diagnosis than do women, aside from differences in lag time to diagnosis and inattention of the AIDS definition to variations among women.

Disease progression also varies by primary route of HIV transmission. Individuals who become infected through injection drug use survive longer compared with those infected through other modes of HIV transmission, whereas contracting HIV by blood transfusion results in the most rapid death following an AIDS diagnosis. The route of contracting HIV is also related to relative frequencies of AIDS-related illnesses. Men who contract HIV sexually from other men are more likely to develop Kaposi's sarcoma and injection drug users are more likely to develop pneumocystis carinii pneumonia, recurrent bacterial pneumonia and pulmonary tuberculosis.

Differences in transmission routes may also account for most of the differences in opportunistic illnesses between men and women. However, the associations between disease and HIV transmission routes are not well understood, with such factors as primary path of entry into the bloodstream, the volume of HIV transmitted and number of exposures to the virus all potentially mediating HIV infection.

Exercise and nutrition, on the other hand, may slow HIV disease, although there is thus far little empirical support for direct relationships. There is also little evidence that alcohol and other psychoactive substance use play a significant role in HIV infection. The most widely accepted co-factors for HIV infection, although not universally accepted, have been infections with other pathogens.

In particular, the interaction between HIV and other viruses (*i.e.*, herpes viruses) has been considered important. Sexually transmitted pathogens and infectious agents spread through non-sterile preparations of drug-injecting equipment trigger immune responses that can stimulate HIV and activate HIVs replication cycle. Co-infection with other immune-suppressing viruses can also facilitate the progression of HIV. Even worse, multiple infections are synergistic and make prognosis dependant on a chain of unpredictable biomedical events. Repeated exposures to HIV complicate the picture further by multiple strains of the virus with varied properties.

Variation in viral strains occurs because of the drift in molecular composition demonstrated in HIV isolates within and between infected persons. Although these and other factors appear related to HIV progression, no true cofactors for HIV disease have been conclusively established. Potential cofactors of HIV infection tend to co-occur and have inextricable effects.

In addition, exposure to infectious agents that may facilitate HIV disease occurs in different patterns among ethnic groups, sexes and sexual-orientation subgroups. Therefore, associations between potential co-factors and disease progression are open to multiple interpretations, including bi-directional causes and unidentified third variables.

LATER-STAGE HIV INFECTION

Following long periods of asymptomatic infection, any number of general and nonspecific early symptoms may develop. Symptoms of HIV infection include chronic low-grade fever; persistent fatigue, diarrhea lasting at least 2 weeks, rashes or other skin conditions, unintentional weight loss of at least 10 pounds, night sweats and mild infections of the mouth or throat.

The later stages of HIV infection are characterised by severe depletion of T-helper lymphocytes and the onset of specific illnesses. Most clinical manifestations of HIV infection are evident relatively late in the course of disease, occurring only after significant immunologic impairment.

Illnesses that occur late in HIV infection reflect the defective-cell-mediated immunity caused by diminished numbers of T-helper lymphocytes. Similar immune dysfunction is common among cancer patients receiving chemotherapy, patients with certain lymphomas and other malignancies and organ transplant recipients. T-helper lymphocyte counts below 200 cells/mm^3 mark what otherwise would be unexplained significant weight loss, chronic diarrhea, new or persistent outbreaks of genital herpes, skin rashes and infections of the mouth, esophagus and vagina. Over 35 per cent of all HIV-related hospitalisations, 29 per cent of hospital costs and over 35 per cent of HIV-positive hospital inpatient deaths occur among people who become systemically ill but have not yet been diagnosed with AIDS.

Cohorts followed before the widespread availability of antiretroviral medications showed that most people survive between 11 and 12 months after receiving an AIDS diagnosis, less than 11 per cent survive 3 years and yet others are known to have a slow-progressing disease, surviving 15 years and beyond. T-helper cell counts below 200 cells/mm^3 substantially increase risk for developing AIDS-related conditions, with 80 per cent of people developing an AIDS-related illness within 3 years of T-helper cell counts dropping below 200/mm^3. The probability of serious illnesses increases as T-helper lymphocytes decline, with survival times for people with T-helper cell counts below 50 cells/mm^3 being generally less than 1 or 2 years. Several factors appear to predict length of life following AIDS-related symptoms.

Studies have shown that the initial condition leading to an AIDS diagnosis strongly predicts survival. Most consistently, individuals first diagnosed with Kaposi's sarcoma are more likely to survive longer than are people diagnosed with pneumocystis carinii pneumonia, who in turn survive longer than those initially diagnosed with other AIDS-associated illnesses. Rothenberg, Woelfel, et al. found that 72 per cent of patients initially diagnosed with Kaposi's sarcoma survived 1 year and 30 per cent survived 5 years, a substantially greater survival time than is associated with other AIDS-related illnesses. Friedman *et al.* concluded that the role of initial AIDS diagnosis in survival may be attributed to the organ systems involved, the degree of immune suppression that characterises its onset and the effectiveness of available treatments.

Survival time is also associated with characteristics of individuals, among which the sex of the infected person is the most controversial. Research has failed to show that nongynecologic manifestations of HIV infection differ between men and women and there are no known sex differences in AIDS prognosis or in the rate of disease progression from HIV infection to AIDS.

Thus, although early explanations for findings of women surviving shorter periods of time tended to stress potential biological co-factors, such as genetics or hormones, sociocultural factors now offer the best explanation for women surviving with AIDS for a shorter time. Men with HIV infection are diagnosed earlier, receive better medical care and have stronger social support networks than do women and those differences likely account for variations in survival.

A history of using injection drugs also contributes to an earlier death for women with AIDS. Sex differences in survival also appear related to women historically having less access to adequate health care, including clinical trials for experimental treatments. Ethnicity also predicts AIDS survival. African Americans survive a shorter time with AIDS than do their White counterparts. Ethnic differences in survival may be the result of several factors, including differences in immune functioning, prevalence of co-factors for disease progression and differences in routes of contracting HIV. Ethnic differences in AIDS survival are, however, best accounted for by sociodemographic differences between African Americans and Whites found in study samples. For example, Hogg et al. found that like other diseases, AIDS morbidity and mortality is closely associated with income level.

Interpreting survival studies, however, requires close attention to their methodological limitations. For example, early studies conducted in New York City demonstrated survival times substantially longer than those reported in

San Francisco cohorts. It was at first thought that the difference reflected relative numbers of gay men versus injection drug users in the respective cohorts. Differences in survival, however, have been accounted for by data management strategies.

Finally, there are problems in trying to compare different survival studies, not only because AIDS has been defined differently over the course of the epidemic, but also because treatment has changed over time.

Later stages of HIV infection are the result of a progressive depletion of the immune system. Loss of T-helper lymphocytes directly and indirectly impairs immune functioning over long clinically asymptomatic periods. Although studies show that some demographic and risk-related characteristics may be related to survival following an AIDS diagnosis, only initial AIDS-defining illnesses have reliably predicted prognosis. Most differences in survival are related to sociocultural factors, particularly access to medical care. Nearer the end of the disease process, people with HIV infection face an array of serious health threats as their immune system declines.

THE AIDS-CASE DEFINING CONDITIONS

Clinical manifestations of HIV-related conditions fall within one of two general classes. Although most conditions result from a depleted immune system, others are a direct result of HIV infection itself, including HIV infection of the lymph nodes, brain, kidneys, abdominal cavity and lungs. Most AIDS-defining conditions, however, result from a deteriorating immune system, including the growth of malignant tumours and development of opportunistic infections that would otherwise be kept in check.

Bartlett identified the 10 most common clinical presentations of HIV infection: persistent lymphadenopathy; pulmonary symptoms suggestive of pneumonia; cytopenia (diminution of blood cells); fungal infections; constitutional symptoms including persistent fever and diarrhea; weight loss; bacterial infections; tuberculosis; persistent symptoms of sexually transmitted diseases; and nervous system disorders. The first formal diagnostic criteria were established in 1982 as a result of early clinical experiences with men who contracted HIV infection through homosexual activity.

The diagnosis was updated in 1985 and again in 1987 to include additional indicator diseases that characterised the diversity of HIV-infected persons. The 1987 case definition for adults and adolescents consisted of 23 clinical diseases. The case definition for children differed from adults by including recurrent bacterial infections and pulmonary problems among indicator diseases and by not considering children under 15 months old with HIV antibodies to be HIV infected because of passive perinatal transfer of maternal antibodies.

The CDC AIDS case definition was once again expanded in 1993. In reference to the conditions included in the diagnosis of AIDS, the CDC stated that "the objectives of these changes are to simplify the classification of HIV infection, to reflect current standards of medical care for HIV infected persons and to categorise more accurately HIV-related morbidity".

The revised case definition also addresses several criticisms of previous diagnostic criteria, such as failure to include manifestations of HIV common among women. The CDC case definition retains the 23 conditions included in the previous diagnosis and adds three new diseases: pulmonary tuberculosis, recurrent pneumonia and invasive cervical cancer. Pulmonary tuberculosis (TB) was added because HIV-induced immune suppression increases the likelihood of activating latent TB.

Recurrent pneumonia was added to the case definition because of the prevalence of bacterial pneumonia, with as much as a fivefold increase among HIV-infected injection drug users compared with their non-HIV-infected counterparts. Finally, invasive cervical cancer was added to the revised case definition because as many as 22 per cent of HIV-infected women present signs of early cervical disease. The major change in the 1993 AIDS case definition was the inclusion of immunologic diagnostic criteria. Unlike previous AIDS diagnoses, the definition specifies that individuals who are asymptomatic but receive an accurate, although not necessarily most recent, T-helper lymphocyte cell count below 200 cells/mm^3 in conjunction with HIV infection meet the criteria for diagnosis with AIDS.

Immune dysfunction is included in the new case definition because immunologic markers are associated with disease progression and used as clinical prognostic indicators. Another reason for including an immunologic marker independent of specific illnesses is that T-helper cell counts carry similar meaning among subgroups of infected persons who may vary in illness presented, some of which may not yet be listed in the case definition.

Finally, people with suppressed immune systems who did not yet have a case-defining illness became eligible for disability benefits. A substantial increase in the number of diagnosed AIDS cases occurred as a result of the expanded 1993 definition. The increase was due to the sudden inclusion of individuals with T-helper counts below 200 cells/mm^3 among persons living with AIDS.

Of the 35,779 AIDS cases reported in the first quarter of 1993, 60 per cent were based on criteria from the expanded definition, with the majority resulting from criteria related to suppressed T-helper lymphocyte counts. Nearly half of all AIDS cases in 1993 were attributed to the T-helper cell criteria. According to the CDC, if all of the estimated one million HIV-infected persons in the United States were to obtain T-helper cell counts, as many as 120,000 to 190,000 would have less than 200 cell/mm^3 but would not yet have had an AIDS-defining illness.

Each AIDS-defining condition entails its own disease processes and implications for prognosis. The majority of AIDS cases have been initially diagnosed with pneumocystis carinii pneumonia. Numerous other AIDS-defining conditions are rare and do not typically occur as initial diagnoses. The signs, symptoms and complications of each condition pose substantially different challenges for people living with AIDS. Immune suppression can mean multiple, simultaneous illnesses.

The manifestations of HIV infection represent a wide spectrum of diseases and a multitude of problems for infected persons. Mental health professionals, of course, are not in a position or role to diagnose or treat these ailments. However, professionals who provide services to clients with HIV infection should be aware of the symptoms, course and potential outcomes of each illness. Below is a brief description of the AIDS-case-defining conditions and other diseases that commonly confront people living with HIV infection.

HIV wasting syndrome is an AIDS-defining condition. Although several disease processes affect the gastro-intestinal system and cause chronic, persistent, disabling loss of weight and body mass, HIV itself can directly cause these symptoms. Diagnosis is determined by involuntary loss of at least 10 per cent of body weight along with either chronic diarrhea or chronic weakness and fever over the course of 30 days, in the absence of other illnesses that could otherwise explain these symptoms. This syndrome is also associated with severe weight loss are symptoms of fatigue, lethargy and physical weakness.

HIV-related neurological disease

Mild to moderate cognitive, affective and motor dysfunctions can occur in HIV infection, with individuals at later stages of AIDS more often experiencing such symptoms. Subtle signs of dysfunction, however, can appear earlier in the course of HIV infection. Early signs of HIV-related neurological disease include difficulty maintaining concentration, memory problems and motor disturbances, including slowing of arm, leg and eye movements.

HIV-related neurological disease is usually diagnosed when symptoms become moderate to severe and disrupt occupational, basic self-care, intellectual, social, or motor functioning. HIV-related neurological disease is caused by the toxic effects of HIV infection of the brain. Clinical symptoms are almost always caused by diffuse brain damage. Neurological effects of HIV infection occur in as many as 90 per cent of HIV-infected individuals, although functional impairment ranges from none to profound.

Viral infections

Cytomegalovirus is a herpes virus and is a very common cause of disease in HIV infection, with a majority of people with AIDS developing some form of active CMV infection. Cytomegalovirus can cause pneumonia, vaginal infection, hepatitis, encephalitis and colitis. However, the most common manifestations are CMV retinitis, CMV esophagitis and CMV colitis. Among the most distressing manifestations of CMV infection is retinitis, which threatens the vision of a significant number of people with AIDS. Irreversible loss of visual acuity and blindness often result from untreated CMV retinitis.

Almost all patients who develop CMV retinitis have T-helper lymphocyte counts below 50 cells/mm^3, making it a later manifestation of HIV infection. In addition to symptomatic illness, CMV also has immune-suppressing effects of its own, potentially complicating the course of HIV infection. Although CMV infection is difficult to treat, advances in antiviral medications have been effective in managing this condition.

Herpes simplex virus infection

Studies have found that as many as 95 per cent of gay men with AIDS were previously infected with herpes simplex virus. Symptoms of herpes simplex infection include small, painful, erupting blisters. When outbreaks of herpes lesions are persistent for at least 1 month, they constitute an AIDS-defining condition. Herpes simplex virus causes ulcerations of the oral, genital and anal mucous lining. In non-immune-suppressed persons, herpes blisters heal within 3 to 4 weeks of their onset.

People with compromised immune systems, however, may have chronic prolonged lesions lasting months if untreated or unresponsive to treatment. Herpes simplex lesions may occur in the esophagus, causing pain and possibly interfering with swallowing. Pneumonitis, pulmonary infection and encephalitis are also possible manifestations. Finally, like cytomegalovirus, herpes simplex virus is a potential cofactor in the progression of HIV infection.

Epstein-Barr virus and hairy leukoplakia
Epstein-Barr virus is associated with infectious mononucleosis. Among people with HIV infection, Epstein-Barr virus infection also involves hairy leukoplakia, an AIDS-defining condition the symptoms of which include white lesions on the tongue and other areas of the oral cavity. Hairy leukoplakia occurs in 19 per cent of individuals with otherwise asymptomatic HIV infection and more frequently among people with advanced immune suppression. Although hairy leukoplakia may resolve on its own, symptoms are relieved by a number of treatments, including antiviral medications.

Progressive Multifocal Leukoencephalopathy (PML)
Caused by a human papovavirus, progressive multifocal leukoencephalopathy occurs in approximately 2 per cent to 4 per cent of AIDS cases. The papovavirus infects the oligodendrocytes of the brain, cells responsible for producing the myelin sheath that coats and insulates neurons. The neurologic symptoms of PML are usually rapid, progressive and fatal, with the majority of afflicted persons dying within months of symptomatic disease.

Symptoms of PML include changes in mental status, memory and language; headache; seizures; loss of coordinated movements; and other motor disturbances. Neurological deficits are focal, affecting specific functions, in contrast with the diffuse and generalised symptoms of HIV encephalopathy.

Fungal infections
Candida is a fungus that normally exists in the mouth and esophagus. With immune suppression, however, candida often progresses to an active disease. Oral infection with candidiasis is commonly called thrush, usually forming removable white plaques on the surface of the tongue and oral cavity. Plaques may be small or widespread and can alternatively appear as small red areas rather than white patches. For an AIDS diagnosis, candidiasis must involve the esophagus, bronchi, trachea, or lungs, but infection may also occur in other organ systems, including the gastrointestinal system and the female genital tract. Vaginal

candidiasis is among the earliest signs of immune suppression for women with HIV infection, often occurring when T-helper cell counts are still relatively high and causing discomfort and possibly discharge.

Coccidioidomycosis

An infection that occurs after fungus particles are inhaled into the lungs, coccidioidomycosis is among the least frequent AIDS-defining conditions. Dysfunctional T-helper lymphocyte mediated immunity allows active and progressive coccidioidomycosis of both the inside and outside lung. Risk increases in direct proportion to declining T-helper lymphocytes, particularly when cell counts drop below 250 cells/mm^3.

There are two general forms of coccidioidomycosis, primary and chronic. The primary form is an acute self-limiting condition involving only the respiratory system. In contrast, the chronic form of the disease may involve several organ systems. People with severely impaired immune systems are most likely to develop pulmonary disease followed by widespread dissemination. For coccidioidomycosis to allow an AIDS diagnosis, the disease must become disseminated to nonpulmonary organs.

Cryptococcoses

Advanced HIV infection increases susceptibility to cryptococcal infections, affecting as many as 6 per cent to 9 per cent of people with AIDS. Cryptococcal infection tends to occur with severe immune suppression. Although the disease may occur in any organ system and often affects the respiratory system, the most common form of infection is Cryptococcal meningitis presenting with headache, stiff neck, nausea, vomiting, malaise and possible seizures. Other common symptoms include hypersensitivity to light and marked changes in mental status.

Histoplasmosis

Histoplasmosis first occurs through inhaling fungus particles, with infection potentially disseminating to other organ systems. Clinical manifestations of infection include fever, skin rashes, anaemia, lymphadenopathy and involvement of vital organs. Histoplasmosis occurs at varying rates across regions of North America, with the central and south-central United States and Ontario and Quebec Canadian provinces having the most concentrated number of cases. As many as 27 per cent of AIDS patients in these areas develop histoplasmosis, as compared with other regions, where infection is virtually nonexistent.

Pneumocystis carinii pneumonia (PCP)

Prior to the wide-scale use of prophylaxis, active pneumocystis carinii (PCP) occurred in as many as 80 per cent of advanced HIV disease cases. First classified as a protozoan, most authorities now agree that pneumocystis carinii *is* a fungus, although this is not conclusive and the taxonomy remains debated. Pneumocystis carinii exists in the environment and is believed to be universally contracted at young ages through inhalation of fungus particles. However, pneumocystis carinii is only clinically expressed under severe immune suppression, particularly when T-helper lymphocyte cell counts fall below 200 cells/mm^3.

However, children infected with HIV develop PCP at earlier stages of infection. Thus, because almost everyone is exposed to pneumocystis carinii *and* because the fungus is suppressed by cellular immunity mediated by T-helper lymphocytes, it has been the predominant manifestation of AIDS in the United States and the most frequent identifiable cause of AIDS-related death. Pneumocystis carinii pneumonia can present with early and diffuse symptoms, including mild tightness of the chest, chronic fever, fatigue and weight loss.

Respiratory symptoms usually include dry/nonproductive cough and progressive shortness of breath. As the pneumonia progresses, tasks with even limited demands become taxing and exhaustive. Pneumocystis carinii can, although rarely, infect the skin, central nervous system, eyes, abdominal walls, lymph nodes, kidneys, liver and several other organ systems. Thus, although pneumocystis carinii is usually limited to the respiratory system, it can become widely disseminated.

Protozoan infections

Cryptosporidiosis

Infection with cryptosporidiosis occurs after spores of the microorganism are either inhaled or ingested. Cryptosporidia causes chronic diarrhea and is responsible for all diarrhea-related illnesses. In AIDS cases, infection can involve any area of the gastrointestinal tract, but the usual site is the small intestine. The AIDS case definition requires that symptoms of chronic diarrhea caused by cryptosporidia persist for a minimum of one month. Cryptosporidiosis also causes gallbladder disease. Treatment for this infection is extremely limited and symptoms, therefore, are chronic, debilitating and often lethal.

Isosporiasis

Like cryptosporidiosis, this infection strikes the gastrointestinal tract, causing diarrhea, abdominal cramping and weight loss. However, unlike other protozoan infections, effective treatments are available for isosporiasis.

Toxoplasmosis

The intercellular protozoan toxoplasma gondii is the cause of toxoplasmosis, the most common infection of the human central nervous system. Exposure to Toxoplasma gondii occurs principally through contact with cat faces. Immune suppression allows for toxoplasmosis infection because of defective cellular immunity. Between 20 per cent and 47 per cent of people with AIDS who carry toxoplasma gondii eventually develop toxoplasmosis encephalitis.

Manifestations usually include a mixture of focal and generalised neurological symptoms, including disturbances in thought processes, lethargy, confusion, memory and language deficits and motor disturbances. Although toxoplasma gondii can infect vital organ systems outside of the central nervous system, a disseminated course of infection is atypical even among HIV-infected persons.

Malignancies

The occurrence of cervical dysplasia in women with HIV infection is related to increased immune suppression. Studies of women who receive organ transplants, however, suggest that progression to cervical cancer may require prolonged periods of immune suppression. Therefore, relatively few cases of invasive cervical cancer have been reported among HIV-infected women. Because invasive cervical cancer usually occurs late in HIV infection and because it has been reported in some HIV-infected women, it was added to the 1993 AIDS case definition following controversy about previous exclusion of conditions related to AIDS in women. Inclusion of invasive cervical cancer as an AIDS-defining condition was also meant to emphasize "the importance of integrating gynaecologic care into medical services for HIV infected women. Early detection of cervical cancer is possible with pap smears, which should be a regular part of health care for HIV-positive women.

HIV-related lymphomas

Non-Hodgkin's-disease lymphomas were among the earliest recognised manifestations of HIV infection. Unlike other lymphomas, those related to HIV infection tend to progress rapidly and have extremely poor prognoses. Although most non-HIV-infected lymphomas involve disease contained to the lymph nodes, HIV lymphomas are distinguished by their widespread involvement of vital organs.

Approximately 26 per cent of HIV-related lymphomas involve the gastrointestinal system, 25 per cent bone marrow, 12 per cent liver, 9 per cent kidneys and 9 per cent lungs. Most common, however, is central nervous system involvement, occurring in 25 per cent to 32 per cent of HIV-related cases of lymphoma and only rarely in non-HIV lymphomas. Symptoms of central nervous system lymphoma include seizures, localised neurologic dysfunction and headache. HIV-related lymphoma usually occurs late in infection, after other AIDS-related conditions have occurred and when T-helper lymphocyte counts drop below 50 cells/mm^3.

Kaposi's sarcoma

Although rare before the HIV epidemic, Kaposi's sarcoma has been the most common malignancy among people with AIDS, with the majority of cases occurring among men who sexually contracted HIV from other men. Homosexually infected men are 20,000 to 40,000 times more likely to develop Kaposi's sarcoma than same-age HIV-negative men. Relatively few cases of Kaposi's sarcoma have occurred among injection drug users and only 2 per cent of cases have an initial diagnosis of Kaposi's sarcoma.

Kaposi's sarcoma typically develops as a mass on the skin, mucous membranes, or internal organs. The disease is usually first noted by skin lesions that appear as dark red-to-violet-coloured areas on light-skinned persons and black or brown lesions on dark-skinned persons. Lesions commonly first occur near the head and neck, as well as on the inside of the mouth. It is also common for Kaposi's sarcoma to afflict internal organs, with 20 per cent to 50 per cent of cases involving the lungs. Thus, the lethality of Kaposi's sarcoma is entirely dependant on the site of disease. In most cases, however, Kaposi's sarcoma has an aggressive and unpredictable course.

People who have Kaposi's sarcoma are likely to later develop opportunistic infections and other malignancies. There has, however, been a steady decline in the number of Kaposi's sarcoma cases observed in recent years among people with AIDS.

Bacterial infections

Mycobacterium diseases

Mycobacterial infections include mycobacterium TB, mycobacterium avium complex and other disseminated mycobacteria. It is estimated that between 4 per cent and 40 per cent of people with AIDS in the United States have active TB and that up to 40 per cent of individuals with active TB are HIV infected. The scenario is even worse in developing counties, with the number of cases of TB in sub-Saharan Africa doubling in recent years.

In some South African countries, nearly one third of HIV infections present clinically with TB as their first manifestation. Mycobacterial TB is contracted person-to-person through respiratory routes of transmission, posing a highly alarming chance for spread. Active mycobacterial TB occurs relatively early in HIV infection, usually with T-helper lymphocyte cell counts between 500 and 200 cells/

mm^3. Tuberculosis can become disseminated to a number of organ systems, with less than half of all TB cases in AIDS being confined to the respiratory system. The course of TB in people with AIDS is typically aggressive, particularly when it remains untreated.

Symptoms may include fever, night sweats, fatigue, malaise and weight loss. When TB is pulmonary, symptoms will usually include persistent cough, production of sputum and chest pain. Pulmonary disease occurs in 70 per cent to 90 per cent of HIV-infected individuals with TB. However, antituberculosis drugs are highly effective when used properly.

Unfortunately, as the TB epidemic has escalated, several multiple-drug-resistant strains of mycobacterium TB have emerged. Thus, HIV infection and TB reciprocally complicate each other's disease processes: persons with HIV are at greater risk of developing TB, standard medical interventions for TB are less effective in HIV-infected persons and TB may be more infectious in persons with HIV infection.

In addition to mycobacterium TB, mycobacterium avium complex (MAC) is common in HIV infection. Although discussed as a single disease, MAC consists of two closely related organisms, mycobacterium avium and mycobacterium intracellular, with mycobacterium avium being the more frequently occurring. These mycobacterium are contracted through contaminated soil, food, water and air-borne water droplets. Cases of MAC have increased each year of the HIV epidemic. Disseminated MAC infection usually occurs late in HIV infection, typically with T-helper lymphocyte counts below 100 cells/mm^3. Clinically, MAC presents as diffuse symptoms of infection that include fever, weight loss, malaise, severe anaemia, anorexia and a number of possible gastrointestinal symptoms, including chronic diarrhea, abdominal pain and malabsorption. Disseminated MAC infection is often lethal among people with AIDS. Unfortunately, there are few effective treatments available for MAC infections, although there have been many advances in preventive and therapeutic medications.

Recurrent bacterial pneumonia

Pneumonia caused by any one of nine different bacteria are frequently seen in people with HIV infection. Bacterial pneumonia was observed early in the HIV epidemic and pulmonary infections have contributed substantially to HIV-related deaths, with as many as 10 per cent of pneurnonias in AIDS patients the result of community-acquired bacterial infections. The onset of bacterial pneumonia is typically abrupt and the duration can last several days, making it distinguishable from the insidious onset and persistent symptoms of pneumocystis carinn pneumonia.

Pneumonia caused by bacteria in HIV-infected persons has a course of disease similar to that found among immune-competent individuals, including persistent fever, productive cough, dyspnea (laboured or difficult breathing) and chest pain. However, unlike people with functional immune systems, symptoms of pneumonia in HIV infection persist for long periods of time. Recurrent bacterial pneumonia is now an AIDS-defining condition.

Non-pneumonia-causing bacterial infections

Compromised immune systems increase susceptibility to a wide range of bacterial infections. The most common infections associated with HIV involve the gastrointestinal system, skin, meninges and sinuses. Bacterial infections tend to occur early in immune suppression, reflecting the aggressive disease-causing capabilities of bacteria in even relatively healthy people.

Recurrent salmonella infection occurs frequently and early in HIV infection and is an AIDS-defining condition. More than 50 per cent of cases of salmonella infection cause severe diarrhea and nearly half involve febrile illness: high fevers that may result in seizures. Salmonella infection in HIV infection is most likely to recur because of incomplete elimination of the disease during what would usually be adequate treatment. The bacteria are also likely to become resistant to treatments following recurrent use.

Sinusitis is another common bacterial infection that is persistent when it occurs among HIV-infected persons.

Caused by as many as four different bacteria, symptoms of sinusitis include fever, headache and upper respiratory distress. Symptoms are most chronic among people with T-helper lymphocyte counts below 200 cells/mm^3. Additional bacterial infections common to HIV infection include oral infections such as gingivitis and periodontitis, both of which can be progressive and painful. Other frequent bacterial infections are sexually transmitted diseases. Pelvic inflammatory disease resulting from gonorrhoeal infection becomes persistent and aggressive in HIV-infected women. Syphilis also takes an aggressive course in HIV infection and includes an increased risk of neuro-syphilis. HIV infection further complicates syphilis by speeding up its course and reducing the effectiveness of antibiotic treatments. Thus, similar to other bacterial infections, co-infection of HIV and sexually transmitted bacteria poses specific problems not encountered when bacterial infections occur in people with functional immune systems.

Virtually any infection or malignancy that is normally suppressed by immune responses can become a complication of HIV infection. For example, although only three cancers are included as AIDS case-defining conditions (non-Hodgkin's lymphoma, Kaposi's sarcoma and invasive cervical cancer), HIV infection is associated with Hodgkin's disease, melanoma and cancers of the colon, lung and testes. Numerous viral, protozoan, fungal and bacterial infections that are usually managed by immune responses frequently cause serious illness.

Manifestations of HIV infection result from interactions among several defects in the protective immune system resulting from interference with and destruction of T-helper lymphocytes. Thus, as HIV infection progresses, disease-causing agents that are usually either completely suppressed or easily managed by immunity become potentially life threatening. Serious immune suppression is also likely to result in simultaneous infections and malignancies that require multiple medical interventions. For these reasons, medical treatments that slow the loss of T-helper lymphocytes, prevent malignancies, or protect against opportunistic infections have been the principal means of combating HIV infection.

BIOMEDICAL INTERVENTIONS

People with HIV infection live longer today than at any other time in the history of the HIV epidemic and can expect to live even longer in the future. Advances in the medical management of HIV disease are constantly emerging. Treatments for HIV infection and its associated complications generally fall into three categories: interventions directed at impeding the progress of HIV, prevention and treatment of opportunistic illnesses and complementary treatments.

Antiretroviral therapies

As the HIV selectively eliminates the branch of the immune system that recognises antigens and coordinates immune responses, antiretroviral treatments act entirely on their own to suppress HIV, HIV's cycle provides points of potential attack on HIV. For example, tat, one of HIV's regulatory genes, is essential for the synthesis of proteins used for HIV production.

A drug that inhibits the activity of the tat gene disrupts the HIV replication cycle and stops production of HIV in chronically infected as well as newly infected cells. Several tat inhibitors have demonstrated some effectiveness in clinical trials and show promise as a future treatment. Drugs that inhibit reverse transcriptase, the enzyme necessary for HIV activation, interfere with the transcription phases of virus production. Reverse transcriptase inhibitors have been the most widely developed and studied antiretroviral medications. Reverse transcriptase is necessary for the replication of HIV and is not found in non-HIV-infected cells. Thus, inhibiting reverse transcriptase does not interfere with normal cell functioning.

Viral replication is interrupted by the drug when RNA is transcribed to DNA. A nucleic acid from the antiretroviral drug is incorporated into the RNA-DNA transcription process, causing a termination in the chain of nucleic acids. Reverse transcriptase inhibitors, however, only suppress

HIV replication in newly infected cells. Once HIV is established in a cell, the effects of reverse transcriptase inhibitors become limited. The first approved and most widely used reverse transcriptase inhibitor is zidovudine (AZT), a drug first developed in the 1960s to treat murine retroviruses.

Numerous studies have shown that zidovudine is effective in slowing HIV progression for most people treated. Effects of zidovudine treatment include increased numbers of T-helper lymphocytes, decreased HIV activity, reduced frequency and severity of opportunistic illnesses and improved general health status. There is also evidence that AIDS is delayed by zidovudine. Zidovudine appears to extend survival for some people with AIDS.

Moore, Hidalgo, Sugland and Chaisson showed that survival with AIDS has increased substantially since 1987 and zidovudine therapy was attributed with much of the improvement. People with AIDS treated with zidovudine demonstrate greater longevity than those who, for what ever reason, did not receive treatment. Zidovudine has its greatest effects when started within 1 year of receiving an AIDS diagnosis. Zidovudine is typically initiated when T-helper lymphocyte counts fall between 200 and 500 cells/mm^3. Early use of zidovudine, before the onset of overt immune suppression or opportunistic illnesses, has been recommended but controversial.

Some patients treated before the onset of AIDS survive longer after an AIDS diagnosis when compared with people not treated early in the course of infection. Antiretroviral therapy is tolerated best when a person is generally healthy because zidovudine is highly toxic for people with advanced immune suppression. However, results from clinical trials show that the maximum benefits of zidovudine are time limited and there is disagreement about exactly when treatment should be initiated. It is generally recommended that antiretrovirals be started when T-helper counts drop below 200 cells/mm^3.

There are a number of limitations associated with zidovudine therapy. Zidovudine may slow down the replication of HIV, but it will not prevent persistent infection. People treated with zidovudine, particularly at high doses, are vulnerable to early side effects that result from its toxicity, including headache, insomnia, nausea, vomiting, abdominal pain, diarrhea, fatigue, rashes, muscle pain and fever. However, most side effects resolve within 8 weeks. The most threatening adverse effect of zidovudine is bone marrow suppression, causing anemia and other potentially serious conditions. Bone marrow suppression therefore leads to immediate discontinuation of zidovudine treatment. Prolonged use of zidovudine, particularly when started early in HIV infection, can result in long-term, often irreversible side-effects.

Zidovudine toxicity is directly related to dose and adjustments often relieve adverse symptoms. Also related to toxicity are the possible teratogenic effects on pregnancy, although they have not yet been fully determined. Expectations of potential adverse effects of zidovudine are among the most common reasons for refusing treatment.

Three additional reverse-transcriptase-inhibiting drugs have been developed and tested: Dideoxycytidine (ddC), Dideoxyinosine (ddC) and 3'-Deoxythmidine-2'-ene (d4T). Each functions similarly to zidovudine by inhibiting the action of reverse transcriptase and therefore interfering with HIV replication. The antiretroviral actions of ddC are increased when taken in combination with zidovudine. Unfortunately, ddC also has toxic side effects, including peripheral neuropathy (numbness, tingling, or pain in the hands and feet), oral ulcerations and skin rashes. Similarly, ddI presents problems with peripheral neuropathy, diarrhea and pancreatitis.

Although d4T has not been as fully tested, it has shown promise as an antiretroviral treatment, although it too has potential adverse effects. Other antiretroviral treatments are under development and may effectively inhibit reverse transcription with lower levels of toxicity.

For example, phosphonosformate (foscarnet) is an effective antiviral drug used to treat herpes viruses, particularly cytomegalovirus, that also has antiretroviral properties. Foscarnet exerts an inhibitory effect against viral enzymes that are important in HIV replication, without interfering with normal cell enzymes. Foscarnet, however, requires intravenous administration and can have many toxic effects. Advances in antiretroviral medications have been most promising in the area of combination therapies. Concurrent use of two or more treatments, or convergent combination therapy, may increase effectiveness and prohibit HIV resistance to these medications.

Combination therapies have potential for future developments in treating AIDS because new drugs are constantly appearing in clinical trials and because when given in the right combination, they may create an effect greater than any single drug. Treatments targeted to other points of the HIV replication cycle have, unfortunately, been less successful at slowing down HIV infection.

Other treatments include drugs that inhibit proteins necessary for the production of regulatory genes specific to HIV and drugs that inhibit cellular enzymes important in HIV production. For example, a new group of drugs that inhibit protease, an enzyme that is essential for HIV replication, has shown efficacy in clinical trials. These drugs bind with the protease enzyme, interfering with its usual functions. It appears that protease inhibitors can effectively slow HIV progression with few toxic side effects and may synergise with zidovudine, ddI, ddC, or d4T.

Promising HIV treatments like protease inhibitors have accelerated government approval procedures for life-threatening illnesses and reach the stage of clinical trials much more rapidly than almost any other treatment in medical history. At any given time, there are hundreds of investigational drug trials for HIV infection and AIDS.

Most manifestations of HIV infection involve opportunistic infections and malignancies that are usually protected against by T-helper lymphocytemediated immunity. Prevention of opportunistic illnesses results in sustained illness-free periods for people with HIV infection. Because many opportunistic illnesses were rare before the HIV epidemic, there has been a rush to establish prophylactic and treatment guidelines.

For example, guidelines for prophylaxis against pneumocystis carinii pneumonia (PCP) include actions to prevent an initial episode of pneumonia, primary prophylaxis, where individuals with T-helper lymphocyte cell counts below 200 cells/mm^3 routinely begin treatment with anti-PCP drugs. Dapsone, bacterium and aerosolised pentamidine are effective in preventing primary and secondary episodes of PCP.

Prophylaxis has also been established for toxoplasmosis encephalitis and mycobacterial infections. Antiviral drugs are widely used to control recurrent symptoms of herpes viruses and members of other virus families. Interferons have been effective in treating Kaposi's sarcoma. Additional advantages are offered by some prophylactic agents because they frequently guard against multiple opportunistic illness. For example, TMP-SMX, used as a PCP preventive, also helps protect against other diseases, including toxoplasmosis. Standards of care are also in place for preventing HIV-related malignancies. In addition to prevention, treatments are available to manage several opportunistic illnesses. Most treatments effective in dealing with diseases in the context of a functional immune system do so in conjunction with cell-mediated immunity.

Unfortunately, as the immune system deteriorates the effectiveness of opportunistic-illness interventions requires greater doses and more time to achieve equal effectiveness. This is problematic in and of itself because many treatments have adverse side effects with prolonged use, particularly in immune-compromised individuals. Another limitation is the potential for resistance to treatments over time, as has been the case with some strains of HIV and several bacteria. It is important to note that advances in the treatment of HIV-related diseases develop rapidly.

New treatments are the product of converging areas of medicine including, but not limited to infectious diseases, immunology, oncology, hematology, neurology and pharmacology. As treatment approaches from different disciplines emerge, they are likely to be combined into promising new therapeutic avenues.

Treatments for HIV infection and related illnesses that have not yet gone through rigorous approval processes are often sought by HIV-infected people. Searching for unconventional treatments when faced with a chronic, life-threatening disease is often an outgrowth of disillusionments and frustrations with traditional medicine. Although initially considered alternatives to standard medical care, unapproved treatments are now referred to as complementary therapies because they are not necessarily replacements as much as they are adjuncts to mainstream treatments. Complementary therapies have become part of a social activist movement within communities heavily affected by AIDS.

Complementary therapies intervene at different points along the HIV replication cycle. Among those that are more commonly used are megadoses of vitamin C, which have been shown to have antiretroviral activity against human retroviruses in laboratory studies. Also used is AL-721, a mixture of lipids believed to alter the membrane of T-helper lymphocytes and viral protective envelope proteins, in an effort to disrupt virus-to-cell binding properties. Other presumed antiretroviral agents include Compound Q (a purified root of a Chinese cucumber), hypericin (an herbal tea) and several preparations related to proteins necessary for HIV biosynthesis. In addition to antiretrovirals, several complementary therapies may act as modulators of the immune system (*e.g.*, naltrexone and disulfiram).

Most of these agents showed early promise but have not stood up to rigorous scientific testing. These treatments are acceptable to traditionalists only to the extent that they do not interfere with standard medical care.

Although complementary treatments can involve holistic and naturalistic approaches, there are invasive procedures that have not yet demonstrated effectiveness but are nonetheless undertaken by many HIV-infected patients. There are several potential risks associated with complementary therapies. First, many complementary approaches have serious adverse effects, such as AL-721, which can cause abdominal pain, nausea and increased cholesterol. Second, it is likely that many of these agents result in immune stimulation or immune suppression, either of which can interact in unpredictable and dangerous ways with HIV infection and traditional medications. Finally, the use of complementary therapies may prohibit individuals from participating in standard medical care and AIDS clinical trials. People with HIV infection who are considering complementary treatments should be advised by a physician about their use.

The costs of AIDS in terms of lives and human resources are immeasurable. The majority of people with AIDS are in the most productive years of their lives. Potential years of life lost because of AIDS is disproportionate among subgroups, particularly ethnic minorities.

The cost of care for HIV infection is catastrophic. Using 15 months as a typical survival time following an AIDS diagnosis, the lifetime cost of the drug zidovudine is over $2,200. Aerosol pentamidine, a prophylactic against Pneumocystis carinii pneumonia, costs over $2,000 per year. Thus, the cost of medical care for an AIDS patient is estimated as high as $147,000. Although some people with HIV infection have private health insurance, the majority rely on public assistance. People with HIV infection will increasingly need public funds as insurance companies require HIV testing prior to accepting new policies.

As the number of HIV infections increases and as people with HIV continue to live longer, there will be increasingly more HIV-positive patients in need of care. These two patterns, more people becoming HIV infected and infected individuals living longer, promise to continue over the next several years. There is great potential for people with AIDS to become burdened by treatment needs. Growing numbers of people with HIV infection live in poverty. Inner-city minorities are less likely to receive early interventions than are their nonminority counterparts and have less access to standard medical treatments for HIV, such as zidovudine and prophylaxis against pneumocystis carinii pneumonia.

SELECTED READINGS

Miller, R. L., Holmes, J. M., & Auerbach, M. I. (1992, August), *"Volunteer experiences of providing AIDS-related educational services"*. Paper presented at the 100th Annual Convention of the American Psycho-logical Association, Washington, DC.

Miller, J. E. (1983), Coping with chronic illness. In J. F. Miller (ed.), *Coping with chronic illness: Overcoming powerlessness.* Philadelphia: Davis.

Ostrow, D., Joseph, J., Kessler, R., Soucy, J., Tal, M., Eller, M., Chmiel, J., & Phair, J. (1989), "Disclosure of HIV antibody status: Behavioural and mental health correlates". *AIDS Education and Prevention.*

Ozawa, M., Auslander, W., & Slonim-Nevo, V. (1993), "Problems in financing the care of AIDS patients". *Social Work.*

Padian, N. S., (1988), "Preventing the heterosexual spread of AIDS". *Journal of the American Medical Association,* 1879.

Pfeiffer, N. (1992, October), "Long term survival and HIV disease: The role of exercise and CD4 response in HIV disease". *AIDS Patient Care.*

Potts, M., Anderson, R., & Baily, M. C. (1991), Slowing the spread of human immunodeficiency virus in developing countries. *Lancet.*

Rosenberg, M. J., Holmes, K. K., & the World Health Organization working group on Virucides. (1993), "Virucides in prevention of HIV infection: Research priorities". *Sexually Transmitted Diseases.*

Schwartzberg, S. S. (1993), "Struggling for meaning: HIV-positive gay men make sense of AIDS". *Professional Psychology: Research and Practice.*

Sikkema, K. J., Kalichman, S. C., Kelly, J. A, & Koob, J. J. Group intervention to improve coping with AIDS-related bereavement: Moel development and an illustrative clinical example, *AIDS Care.*

Somlai, A., & Kalichman, S. (1994, August) *The spiritual practices and needs of people living with HIV-AIDS.* Paper presented at the 102nd Annual Convention of the American Psychological Association, Los Angeles.

Sweeney, J., Peters, B. S., & Main, J. (1991), "Clinical care and management". *AIDS Care.*

Taerk, G., Gallop, R. M., Lancee, W. J., Coates, R. A., & Fanning, M. (1933), "Recurrent themes of concern in groups for health care professionals". *AIDS Care.*

Slowinski, J. W. (1989, September), "Psychological needs of HIV-positive and AIDS patients". *Medical Aspects of Human Sexuality.*

8

HIV Transmission through Breast-feeding

Strategies to reduce child mortality and to promote family health have resulted in considerable improvements in child health, in the past three decades. Promotion of breast-feeding has played an important role since breast-feeding contributes to reduced mortality by providing optimum nutrition, by protecting against common childhood infections and by its child-spacing effects. However, the emergence of HIV threatens to reverse gains in child health, since children are at risk of acquiring HIV infection through transmission from an HIV-infected mother. It is recognized that breast-feeding by an HIV-infected mother increases the risk of HIV transmission to her infant.

Since the beginning of the HIV pandemic, approximately three million children under 15 years of age worldwide have been infected with HIV and current estimates suggest that 600,000 children are newly infected annually. The majority of these children live in sub-Saharan Africa, where between 25-40 per cent of HIV-Infected children die before their fifth birthday and HIV is already contributing to increased childhood mortality. Although HIV transmission through breast-feeding is only partially responsible for this increase, HIV and infant feeding is an important public health issue, particularly in regions where HIV prevalence is high and infectious diseases and malnutrition are the leading causes of childhood death. Countries need to develop sound policies regarding the prevention of HIV transmission through breast-feeding while continuing to protect, promote and support breast-feeding for infants of HIV-negative women and women of unknown serostatus.

MOTHER-TO-CHILD TRANSMISSION

Mother-to-child transmission of HIV, which can occur during pregnancy, delivery or breast-feeding, is responsible for more than 90 per cent of HIV infection in children worldwide. Both HIV type 1 (HIV-1) and HIV type 2 (HIV-2) can be transmitted from mother to child, but HIV-2 is transmitted much less frequently, as it is less pathogenic than HIV-1. The remaining 10 per cent of paediatric infections are attributed to transfusion with contaminated blood and blood products, use of contaminated medical equipment, other practices that cut or pierce the skin, or sexual contact. Most children acquire the virus through transmission from an HIV-Infected mother, therefore, the incidence of paediatric HIV reflects that of HIV infection in women of child-bearing age.

Mother-to-child transmission (MTCT) of HIV focuses attention on women, but the use of the term MTCT is not to imply blame, whether or not a woman is aware of her own infection status. A woman can acquire HIV through unprotected sex with an infected partner, by receiving contaminated blood, or through exposure to unsterile instruments or medical procedures. HIV is often introduced into the family through the woman's sexual partner, often the father of her child. The prevalence of HIV varies considerably from region to region.

Women and children in sub-Saharan Africa are disproportionately affected, with eight in every 10 HIV-infected women worldwide and nine in every 10 newly infected children living in this region. In West and Central Africa, HIV prevalence in pregnant women currently reaches 10-15 per cent in some urban areas and 1-5 per cent in others. Prevalences in East Africa are higher at 15-25 per cent in urban areas and 5-10 per cent in rural areas, while in Southern Africa antenatal seroprevalences of 20-30 per cent and in some places even as high as 40 per cent, have been reported.

In the Caribbean, Central America and South America, HIV-1 seroprevalence rates currently range from 0.1 per cent to 5.0 per cent. Asia is experiencing a rapidly growing epidemic with seroprevalence rates in big cities of Cambodia, India and Thailand currently ranging from 1-5 per cent.

Rates of mother-to-child transmission

Estimates of the rate of mother-to-child transmission of HIV in cohorts of women who have not received any preventive treatment range from 15-25 per cent in industrialized countries to 25-45 per cent in developing countries. The highest rates of MTCT have been found in women in Africa. Differences in study methods, the composition of the populations studied and the prevalence of cofactors of transmission may explain some of these differences. However, it is likely that much of the increased rate of transmission seen in women in sub-Saharan Africa is associated with breast-feeding, where many women breast-feed for about 2 years. In an attempt to quantify the relative contribution of intrauterine and intrapartum transmission of HIV in non-breast-fed infants, a working definition of timing has been proposed.

In utero infection

In in utero infection, a child is classified as having been infected during pregnancy (in utero) if HIV-1 genome is detected within 48 hours of delivery by polymerase chain-reaction test (DNA-PCR) or viral culture.

Intrapartum infection

Acquisition of infection is assumed to have occurred during delivery (Intrapartum) if these diagnostic tests were negative in a sample taken during the first 48 hours after delivery, but became positive in subsequent samples taken within 7-90 days of delivery. Following this classification, a French study estimated that of the infants infected with HIV, 35 per cent of the non-breast-fed infants studied were infected before birth and 65 per cent were infected late in pregnancy or during delivery. A recent review indicated that in women who did not breast-feed their infants, about one-third of MTCT infection was acquired during the intrauterine period. In women who did breast-feed their infants, less than a quarter of all MTCT was acquired during the intrauterine period.

Table 1
Percentage HIV infection acquired by different routes

	Partially breast-fed / breast-fed	*Non-breast-fed infants*
During intrauterine period	20%	33%
During delivery	45-50%	67%
Postpartum, by breast-feeding	30-35%	0

Breast-milk transmission of HIV has been well documented. The first reports indicating the possibility of HIV-1 transmission through breast milk were in breast-fed infants of women who were infected postnatally through blood transfusion or through heterosexual exposure.

Higher rates of mother-to-child transmission of HIV are observed where most infants are breast-fed rather than where fewer infants are breast-fed. However, other reasons for variations in transmission rates, such as maternal nutritional status, stage of HIV disease and possible differences in transmission of HIV subtypes cannot be excluded. Additional evidence is provided by results from prospective studies which indicate that among infants born to HIV-infected mothers, those who are breast-fed are more likely to be infected than those who are formula-fed, even allowing for other factors known to be associated with mother-to-child transmission of HIV.

Although HIV has been detected in breast milk, mechanisms of breast-milk transmission are not yet fully understood. The respective roles of cell-free and cell-associated virus in breast-milk transmission are not known, nor is the association between plasma and milk virus levels understood. The portal of entry for the virus via the infant mucosa also merits further investigation. Animal models have been used to explore potential mechanisms of transmission. It is possible to infect neonatal rhesus monkeys with simian immunodeficiency virus and kittens with feline immunodeficiency virus by applying cell-free virus on the mucosa. This suggests that cell-free HIV in breast milk could infect cells of the intestinal mucosa. M-cells, which are specialized epithelial cells found in the Peyer's patches of the intestinal mucosa, may be a mechanism allowing infectious agents such as HIV to cross the intact mucosa. M-cells engulf and transport the pathogen and present it to macrophages that indent the serosal surface of the M-cell. Results from in vitro studies on rabbit M cells suggest that HIV-1 particles could use M cells to cross the intestinal barrier.

A recent in vitro study indicated that HIV-infected cells themselves may also play an important role by stimulating ordinary enterocytes to engulf HIV particles presented by HIV-infected cells in the intestinal lumen. Moreover, HIV RNA has been detected in the oropharyngeal and gastric aspirates of a substantial proportion of infants born to HIV-infected mothers.

Early studies investigating the frequency of breast-milk transmission and associated factors were limited by small numbers as well as by the predominance of one method of infant feeding in any one cohort. In 1992, a meta-analysis was carried out using data from four studies reporting on 42 recently infected women and six studies reporting on 1772 women with established infection. The majority of the women had breast-fed for 2-4 weeks and 106 women had breast-fed for longer than six months. The estimated additional risk of transmission from breast milk, above that occurring during pregnancy and delivery, among women with established HIV infection, was approximately 15 per cent (95 per cent Confidence Interval 7-22 per cent).

However, 15 per cent may be an underestimation among women who breast-feed for longer periods of time. The risk of transmission through breast milk among women with recent infection (HIV infection acquired in the postpartum period) was nearly twice as high (29 per cent (95 per cent 16-42 per cent)). Insufficient information is available to estimate the exact association between duration of breast-feeding and the risk of transmission. However, there is strong evidence for a gradual and continued increase in transmission risk as long as the child is breast-fed.

Transmission of HIV through breast milk can take place at any point during lactation. The persistence of maternal antibodies and the presence of a "window period" during which infection is undetectable using currently available technology, make it impossible to determine whether an infant has been infected during delivery (intrapartum) or through breast-feeding in the period following birth. Therefore, when seropositive women breast-feed their infants, it is not possible to differentiate between HIV transmission attributable to delivery and that resulting from breast-feeding from birth.

Later postnatal transmission through breast-feeding can be determined using currently available diagnostic tools. Studies of infants found to be negative by PCR testing at 2-6 months of age, but who subsequently showed evidence of infection, have provided estimates of the risk of late postnatal transmission (after 3-6 months of age) ranging from 4-12 per cent.

COLOSTRUM AND MATURE MILK

Cell-free and cell-associated HIV-1 have been detected in both colostrum and mature breast milk of women with established HIV infection.

In a study in Haiti, HIV DNA (cell-associated virus) was detected in 70 per cent of 47 colostrum samples and about 50 per cent of breast-milk samples obtained at 6 (n = 30) and 12 (n = 15) months postpartum. HIV DNA was detected in 47 per cent of 129 samples of breast milk collected 15 days after delivery and in 20 per cent of 96 samples collected six months after delivery.

Both studies suggest a higher level of cell associated HIV in early milk compared to later, which would reflect the relatively high level of cells in colostrum compared to mature milk.

Somewhat differently, in a study in Kenya a higher proportion of samples of milk collected between seven days and six months had HIV DNA (65 per cent of 108 breast milk samples) than did colostrum (51 per cent of 77 samples) (p = 0. 05). Among positive samples, the proportion of infected cells ranged from less than 1 in 10 000 cells to 1 in 3. High concentrations of HIV-Infected cells were more common during the period 8-90 days after delivery than in samples taken either earlier or later.

A second study quantified HIV-1 RNA (measuring cell-free virus) from breast-milk supernatants collected from the same group of women at the same times. The range of viral concentration in the breast-milk supernatants was very wide and, although the difference was not statistically significant, viral load tended to be higher in milk collected more than 8 days after delivery than in milk samples taken earlier (p=0.10). The potential effect of various factors makes it difficult to draw any conclusions about the relative risk of transmission through colostrum and mature breast milk. First, colostrum and mature breast milk contain different types of cells and different levels of immune modulating components (e.g. vitamin A, immunoglobulins and lactoferrin). Second, the total volume of colostrum ingested by the infant is much smaller than that of mature breast milk. Third, the infant's immune system is less well developed during the first few days of lactation than in later lactation, while younger infants have an increased blood concentration of maternal antibodies.

The overall risk of mother-to-child transmission is increased by a range of factors related to HIV disease, the mother and the infant. Some of these factors may also affect the risk of transmission through breast milk. Maternal risk factors include indicators of disease progression, such as high viral load, low CD4 count and viral characteristics. The observation that the risk of transmission through breast-feeding is higher if the mother is infected postnatally suggests that the higher viral load associated with recent infection may also increase the risk of breast-feeding transmission. However, it is not clear whether viral load in blood and in breast milk are correlated.

Viral load in the breast milk of postnatally infected women is an area that requires further study. Low CD4 counts have been associated with detection of HIV DNA in breast milk. A Kenyan study found a strong correlation between maternal immuno-suppression (low CD4 counts) and the prevalence and concentration of breast milk HIV-1 DNA. However, knowledge of the role of maternal immuno-suppression and advanced HIV disease in breast-milk transmission remains limited.

In a Malawi study of 338 women with HIV, 196 (58 per cent) of whom were deficient in vitamin A, HIV transmission was significantly associated with vitamin A status, independent of maternal CD4 status. Vitamin A deficiency may increase the risk of mother-to-child HIV transmission by impairing T and B cell function, resulting in increased maternal viral load and reduced antibody concentrations. Alternatively, vitamin A deficiency could be a marker of advanced HIV disease, which may be the cause of the higher observed mother-to-child transmission rate.

In a study of 72 women with CD4 counts of less than 400/ml in Nairobi, vitamin A deficiency was associated with a linear increase in the prevalence of HIV-1 DNA in breast-milk cells. All six women with vitamin-A levels < 20 mg/dl had detectable HIV-1 DNA in their breast milk, compared to only three of eight women with vitamin-A levels at or above 40 mg/dl.

Although the association between vitamin A and HIV in breast milk has been documented, no studies have been published concerning the role of vitamin A deficiency in breast-milk transmission. Vitamin A deficiency in HIV-Infected women has been reported to be associated with fissured nipples, which may facilitate transmission of HIV through breast-feeding. Poor breast-feeding techniques, especially poor attachment of the infant to the breast, may result in fissured nipples and hence HIV transmission may be prevented through breast-feeding counselling and skilled help with positioning and attachment.

HIV has been recovered from vaginal and cervical secretions of pregnant women and from gastric secretions of infants born to HIV-seropositive women. Delivery factors that increase contact between the infant and HIV-infected maternal body fluids (cervico-vaginal secretions and blood) may therefore be the mechanism for increased risk of transmission. Vitamin A deficiency may also be a co-factor for increased risk associated with delivery, through impaired integrity of epithelial surfaces and vaginal viral shedding.

Neonatal skin and mucous membranes are ineffective barriers against infective organisms. Direct invasion of the skin and oral and gastric mucosa by HIV may play a role in transmission from mother to child, including through breast milk. Traumatic or inflammatory disruption of the skin or mucous membranes may further increase the risk of transmission. Disruption of the epithelial integrity of the mucous membranes of the intestine or mouth, caused by nutritional factors or infection, may increase the risk of HIV .transmission through breast milk.

Table 2
Risk factors associated with increased overall risk of mother-to-child transmission

Strong evidence	*Limited evidence*
Maternal	Vitamin A deficiency
High viral load	Anaemia
Viral characteristics	Sexually transmitted disease
Advanced disease	Chorloamnionitis
Immune deficiency	
HIV infection acquired during pregnancy or breast-feeding period	Frequent unprotected sexual intercourse
	Multiple sex partners
	Smoking Injecting drug use
	Smoking
	Injecting drug use
Obstetric	
Vaginal delivery	Invasive procedures
Prolonged rupture of membranes	Epistomy
Infant	
Prematurity	Leisons of skin and/or mucous membranes (oral thrush)
Breast-feeding	

Factors resulting in disruption of the integrity of infants' mucous membranes, such as oral thrush, may be associated with an increased risk of breast-milk transmission. Feeding with cow's milk, allergic reactions to complementary foods and infectious illness can all result in intestinal damage. Because damage to the epithelial integrity of the intestine may facilitate entry of HIV, mixed feeding might be more risky for HIV transmission than exclusive breast-feeding. Infants could thus be doubly disadvantaged by being at risk of HIV transmission through simultaneous exposure to HIV through breast-feeding and the risks related to replacement feeding. Only three studies have compared the rate of transmission in exclusively breast-fed, partially breast-fed and formula-fed infants. Although the highest transmission rate was found in exclusively breast-fed infants, the lowest rate in formula-fed infants and intermediate rates in the mixed-feeding groups, the number of exclusively formula-fed or breast-fed infants in these studies was small and the differences in rates of transmission were not statistically significant.

ANTI-INFECTIVE PROPERTIES OF BREAST MILK IN WOMEN WITH HIV

One of the most important benefits of breast milk is its ability to protect against common childhood infections such as diarrhoea, pneumonia, neonatal sepsis and acute otitis media. It has been assumed, but not proven, that the breast milk of HIV-Infected women also protects infants against these infections. In a study in Kinshasa of 19 infected children, development of clinical AIDS was not associated with two particular types of infant feeding practice.

However, morbidity was significantly higher in 237 non-HIV-infected children (of both infected and uninfected mothers) who were not exclusively breast-fed, compared with 81 uninfected infants who were exclusively breast-fed during the first six months of life. In Durban, South Africa, exclusively breast-fed infected children had a slower rate of progression to AIDS than those on mixed feeds. Two recent studies from South Africa compared partially breast-fed and exclusively formula-fed HIV-infected infants. In these studies, both groups had similar frequencies of failure to thrive, diarrhoea and pneumonia. Uninfected infants of HIV-positive mothers also had a comparable frequency of these conditions, whether they were partially breast-fed or exclusively formula-fed.

However, these results should be interpreted with great-caution since the failure to detect a difference in health outcomes between breast-fed and formula-fed infants may reflect factors specific to these studies. These include: short duration of exclusive breast-feeding and the inclusion of infants that had stopped breast-feeding in the breast-feeding group; a relatively safe environment (water, electricity, sanitation *etc.*) that minimized the risks of formula feeding; and a relatively literate, urban study population with access to continual health care, as part of a research study design. It is unlikely that these findings would be replicated in studies from other settings in sub-Saharan Africa without additional support being given to women who choose not to breast-feed.

All basic forms of immunoglobulins IgG, IgM, IgA, IgD and IgE are present in breast milk. The most abundant is usually secretory IgA. The role of HIV-specific antibodies in breast milk in inhibiting HIV transmission through breast-feeding has been investigated. Breast milk in women with established HIV infection has been found to have HIV-specific IgG, with its wide spectrum of activity against HIV proteins, comparable to HIV-specific IgG in serum.

The spectrum of activity of serum IgA against HIV has been found to be similar to that of serum IgG, but the spectrum of activity of HIV-specific secretory IgA (sIgA) in breast milk is directed against only a limited number of viral proteins (env protein, gp 160, core proteins).

In a study of breast-milk samples from 215 HIV-infected women in Rwanda, the most frequently identified HIV-specific antibody in breast milk was IgG (in >95 per cent of samples), the next was IgM (in 41-78 per cent of samples) and the least frequent was IgA (in 23-41 per cent of samples). Lack of persistence of HIV-specific IgM in breast milk collected at 18 months was associated with a high risk of transmission of HIV. Of 20 children receiving breast milk with detectable HIV DNA in samples collected at day 15, but without detectable IgM in later samples, 47 per cent were infected with HIV. In those with detectable DNA in breast milk samples at day 15 and with IgM in later samples only 30 per cent became infected. This suggests that IgM may protect against breast-milk transmission of HIV.

The rate of transmission was 18 per cent in infants of mothers whose breast-milk sample at day 15 had undetectable HIV DNA, regardless of IgM levels. Other components of breast milk are protective against viral infections. Human lactoferrin has been shown in vitro to have an inhibitory activity against HIV and lipid-dependent antiviral activity directed at HIV and other enveloped viruses and bacteria has also been described.

STRATEGIES TO REDUCE BREAST-MILK TRANSMISSION

The best way to prevent HIV infection of children through mother-to-child transmission, including transmission through breast milk, is to prevent HIV infection of young girls and women of child-bearing age. In sub-Saharan Africa, Asia and the Caribbean the main mode of HIV transmission is heterosexual contact. In industrialized countries, although most women with HIV have a history of injecting drug use (IDU), or sexual partners with a history of IDU or bisexuality, heterosexual transmission is becoming an increasingly important route of infection.

The risk of HIV infection in women is increased by such factors as immaturity of the genital tract, cervical ectopy, sexually transmitted diseases and poor nutritional status. Cultural, social and economic factors also contribute to HIV transmission by increasing the vulnerability of girls and women. Strategies to prevent all mother-to-child transmission of HIV, including through breast-milk, should be linked to primary prevention programmes that provide education about safer sex, condoms and diagnosis and treatment of sexually transmitted diseases and that ensure the safety of medical procedures.

HIV prevention should be emphasized for women who test seronegative in pregnancy because of the particularly high risk of MTCT if mothers are infected with HIV during pregnancy and breast-feeding.

For an HIV-infected woman to eliminate completely the risk of HIV transmission through breast-feeding she needs to feed her infant from birth with suitable replacements for breast milk. Currently there is little information on the safety and feasibility of using breast-milk substitutes in developing countries. Several investigators have attempted to use mathematical models to offer guidance to policy-makers in different settings for weighing the relative risks and benefits of breast-feeding and other infant feeding methods in view of the HIV epidemic. These models are limited by the available data regarding the risks associated with various methods of infant feeding and their inability to consider all the factors that influence decision-making about infant feeding. In particular, although there is much evidence of the benefits of breast-feeding in reducing morbidity and mortality in infants whose mothers are not infected with HIV, currently there is little information regarding the effect of replacement feeding on infant morbidity and mortality for infants whose mothers are HIV-infected.

Where adequate replacement feeding is not possible, mothers may choose among three other strategies to reduce the risk of breast-milk transmission:

- Exclusive breast-feeding followed by early cessation of breast-feeding. Early cessation of breast-feeding may reduce exposure and hence the risk of breast milk transmission, while not eliminating the risk entirely, as the infant remains exposed for the first few months.
- Heat treatment of expressed breast milk
- Wet-nursing by a tested HIV-negative women
- Early cessation of breast-feeding

Early cessation of breast-feeding reduces the risk of HIV transmission by limiting the length of time that an infant is exposed to HIV through breast milk. Women who are not able to provide adequate and hygienic replacement feeding to their infants from birth may consider this option in order to reduce the cumulative risk of longer breast-feeding duration.

In vitro studies have demonstrated that heat treatment of breast milk to which a known quantity of HIV had been added, using the Holder pasteurization method (at 62.5°C for 30 minutes), reduces the infectious titre of cell-free and cell-associated virus by more than five logs and six logs, respectively).

Breast milk contains substances that inhibit infectious agents. Several studies have reported that HIV is inactivated when milk is left to stand at room temperature for half an hour. In the first two of these studies, the inhibitory effects of breast milk were attributed to a milk-lipase-activated factor that released fatty acids which were thought to dissolve or disrupt the viral envelope. Newburg *et al.*, demonstrated that human milk glycosaminoglycans inhibit binding of HIV glycoprotein gp 120 to host cell CD4 receptors. There is a need to evaluate alternatives for treating breast milk, which utilize or enhance the action of naturally occurring anti-HIV factors to prevent breast-milk transmission of HIV.

All strategies to modify or treat breast milk to render it noninfectious would involve expressing milk and some women may find it difficult to sustain this process for long periods of time. This should not prevent the option being offered and professional support should be provided when women choose it. Expression and heat treatment may also be a temporary solution during periods of increased transmission risk, as in cases of cracked nipples or breast abscess and for low-birth-weight or sick infants for whom the risk of artificial feeding is greater. Heat treatment of breast milk is recommended for all milk banks, which should also screen milk donors for HIV.

In communities where wet-nursing by a family member is practised this option can be considered. It will be necessary for the wet-nurse to agree to and understand the implications of voluntary HIV counselling and testing (VCT). She would also have to be counselled about HIV and be able to avoid becoming infected during breast-feeding.

Antiretroviral Therapy

The use of AZT (zidovudine) during the second and third trimester in pregnant women and in infants during the first six weeks of life, in the absence of breast-feeding, can reduce mother-to-child transmission of HIV by two-thirds. A "short course" regimen of AZT (after 36 weeks gestation and without the neonatal component), combined with formula feeding, has recently been shown in Thailand to reduce mother-to-child HIV transmission by half.

The latter approach may be more feasible where women present late for prenatal care, or where health service resources are limited. Further reductions in mother-to-child HIV transmission may be possible with the use of a combination of antiretroviral drugs, which are currently being evaluated in clinical trials in both breast-feeding and non-breast-feeding populations.

The effectiveness of AZT in reducing mother-to-child transmission has been demonstrated only in non-breast-fed infants. It Is currently not known to what extent infants who have escaped infection during pregnancy and delivery, following prophylactic therapy in their mothers with AZT, are at risk of becoming infected subsequently through breast-feeding. However, it is likely that antiretroviral therapy around the time of delivery will not be as effective if the infant is then exposed through breast-feeding.

Since many HIV-infected mothers may face obstacles to replacement feeding—for example stigma, affordability, risk to the infant of other infections and malnutrition—the effectiveness of antiretroviral treatment of breast-feeding mothers/or breast-fed infants, with and without a postnatal treatment component, is an important research question.

Selected Readings

American Academy of Pediatrics Policy Statement. "Breast-feeding and the Use of Human Milk". *Pediatrics*, 1997.

Bridbord K., Willoughby A. "Vitamin A and mother-to-child transmission". *Lancet* 1994.

Dunn DT, Newell ML, Ades AE, Peckham C. "Risk of human immunodeficiency virus type 1 transmission through breast-feeding". *Lancet* 1992.

Datta P, Embree JE, Kreiss JK, *et. al.*, "Mother-to-child transmission of human immunodeficiency virus" type 1: report from the Nairobi study. *Journal of Infectious Diseases*, 1994.

Greenberg BL, Semba RD, Vink P. *et. al.* "Vitamin A deficiency and maternal-infant transmission of HIV in two metropolitan areas in the United States". *AIDS*, 1997.

Nduati R, John GC, Mbori-Ngacha DA, *et. al.*, "Breast disease among lactating HIV-1 infected women". *Xth ICASA*. Abidjan.

Thea DM, Steketee RW, Pliner V. *et. al.*, "The effect of maternal viral load on the risk of perinatal transmission of HIV-1". *AIDS*, 1997.

Thapa S, Short R V, Pott M. "Breast-feeding, birth spacing and their effects on child survival". *Nature* 1989.

9

AIDS: A Challenge for Human Race

A decade after the human immunodeficiency virus (HIV) was first identified as the cause of acquired immune deficiency syndrome (AIDS), the disease has been reported in nearly all developing and industrial countries. In many developing countries the HIV/AIDS epidemic is spreading rapidly. In major cities of Argentina, Brazil, Cambodia, India and Thailand, more than 2 per cent of pregnant women now carry HIV. These levels are similar to those found ten years ago in such African countries as Zambia and Malawi, where more than one in four pregnant women are now infected.

Meanwhile, the disease is spreading rapidly in Asia. In Latin American and the Caribbean countries the number of new infections has been steady at about 200,000 per year for several years, while the countries of eastern Europe and central Asia are experiencing the initial stages of rapid spread. Only in North America and western Europe has the number of new infections declined from its peak in 1986, but even here the future of the epidemic is unclear as it invades lower-income populations whose education and access to health care more closely resemble those of the developing world. AIDS is clearly taking an immense and growing human toll.

Because AIDS kills mostly prime-age adults, it increases the number of children who lose one or both parents; some of these orphans suffer permanent consequences, due to poor nutrition or withdrawal from school. Numbers cannot begin to capture the suffering caused by the disease. AIDS is not alone in causing human suffering, however especially in the developing world.

Given the many other pressing problems, how much time, effort and resources should governments devote to fighting AIDS? Views differ widely. Some people consider AIDS to be a late-twentieth-century version of the Black Death, which devastated Europe in the fourteenth century. According to this view, governments should do everything in their power to slow the epidemic. Others think that governments should do little or nothing, either because they think AIDS will not be a major problem in their country or because they think that governments are powerless to change the private behaviour that spreads the virus.

AIDS is a large and growing problem and that governments can and should actively confront the epidemic. Some policies will be much more effective than others and it distinguishes between activities that can be undertaken by households and the private sector, including non-governmental organisations (NGOs); those that should be initiated by developing country governments; and those that should be most strongly supported by donor governments and the international development community.

HIV is a fatal, sexually transmitted disease (STD). After an initial week or two of flulike symptoms, the disease has no visible effects on the infected person during an asymptomatic period, which can be as short as two years or as long as 20. Although the average time without symptoms is about ten years in industrial countries, limited data suggest that it might be as short as five years among the poorest people in the poorest countries.

Then, in all but a very small proportion of cases, the disease destroys the immune system. This leaves the infected person vulnerable to other infectious diseases, which are typically fatal within six to 24 months. Like other STDs, HIV is difficult to transmit except by sex or other direct contact with the bodily fluids of an infected person. The major modes of transmission are sexual intercourse, reuse of contaminated syringes by injecting drug users, infection via birth or nursing from mother to child, reuse of needles in medical settings and transfusions of contaminated blood or blood products.

About three-quarters of HIV transmission worldwide is through sex. Of these sexual transmissions, about three-quarters involve heterosexual intercourse and one-quarter involve sexual relations between men. In developing countries, sex accounts for an even greater proportion of cases. In sub-Saharan Africa, Asia and the Caribbean, sexual transmission is overwhelmingly between men and women; less than 1 per cent involve homosexual acts. In Latin America and Eastern Europe, however, sex between men still accounted for most sexual transmission as recently as the early 1990s.

The next most important means of transmission after sexual intercourse is the sharing of unsterilised needles among injecting drug users. Transmission through injecting drug use has been the primary mode of transmission in China and Southeast Asia, except in Thailand, where heterosexual transmission has outpaced transmission by needle sharing.

Injecting drug use is also thought to account for about one-quarter to one-third of transmissions in Brazil and Argentina. HIV can spread through a population of injecting drug users extremely rapidly, in some locales infecting the majority within a few months. The importance of mother-to-child transmission varies widely across countries. The major mode of infection among infants can occur in the uterus through contact with the mother's blood at birth or later through breastfeeding. Since mother-to-child transmission can occur only if the mother is herself infected, it is most common in widespread heterosexual epidemics, such as in sub-Saharan Africa.

HIV may also be spread through medical injections. In some of the poorest countries, injections are the preferred delivery system for a variety of medications and the same syringe may be used on many people in one day without sterilisation between injections. However, even in these countries, medical injections with dirty needles are thought to account for less than 5 per cent of all HIV infections.

Transmission through blood transfusions, once a cause for concern in many countries, has been nearly eliminated in many high and middle-income countries by routine screening of blood for transfusions.

In developing countries however, transmission through the blood supply has yet to be eliminated, especially where HIV prevalence rates are high among blood donors and where screening blood for HIV has not yet become routine. But while transmission through transfused blood and other blood products greatly increases the risk of medical care and can rapidly spread HIV among specific populations—for example, among haemophiliacs in industrial countries in the 1980s—HIV transmission through transfusions has never accounted for more than about 10 per cent of total HIV infections, even in developing countries.

The most obvious impact of AIDS is on the expectancy and health. Measuring and predicting these impacts are difficult, not only because of the lack of quality data, but also because the relative size of an impact depends on many factors besides the spread of AIDS, including success in fighting other health problems. Available evidence discussed below suggests that in the most severely affected countries, AIDS threatens to reverse a century of progress in the fight against infectious diseases.

Elsewhere, it is likely to account for an increased share of the infectious disease burden. Even so, AIDS is only one of many health problems confronting people in developing countries. Indeed, the poorer the country, the more likely it is that other problems—including easily treated problems like malnutrition and diarrhoea—account for a large share of the burden of disease.

The proportion of total deaths caused by a disease is an imperfect representation of its burden on society because it ignores illness and does not distinguish among the deaths of people of different ages. Murray and Lopez have estimated the cost of diseases in terms of disability-adjusted life years, or DALYs. Introduced by the World Development Report 1993, a DALY includes the disability as well as the mortality effects of disease and uses age weights to discount the importance of infant and elderly deaths. In 1990, poor health resulted in the loss of about 265 DALYs per thousand persons per year in developing countries, almost twice the 124 DALYs per thousand per year lost in industrial countries.

Since HIV/AIDS deaths entail substantial disability before death and disproportionally strike prime-age adults, HIV/AIDS has a larger impact on health measured as DALYs than when measured as a share of total deaths. However, the difference is not large: Murray and Lopez project that HIV/AIDS would account for almost 3 per cent of all DALYs lost in developing countries in the year 2020, up from 0.8 per cent in 1990. One reason that HIV/AIDS does not account for a larger percentage of lost DALYs is that other causes of death in developing countries also entail substantial disability and premature death.

When we focus attention on infectious disease, the contribution of HIV/AIDS to the disease burden looms larger. Such a focus is particularly relevant to our overarching purpose of identifying the appropriate roles for developing country governments in the fight against AIDS because economic theory, public health teaching and long-standing practice all affirm that governments should play a significant role in preventing the spread of infectious disease. By 2020 infectious diseases, which currently account for about 30 per cent of deaths and one-quarter of lost DALYs in developing countries, will have declined to about 14 per cent of both measures. But the contribution of HIV/AIDS to the infectious disease burden in developing countries is projected to increase sharply, from about 2 per cent of deaths and 3 per cent of lost DALYs to about 14 per cent of deaths and nearly one-fifth of lost DALYs.

Moreover, because HIV is an increasingly important factor in the spread of TB, it is estimated that about one out of four TB deaths among HIV-negative people in 2020 would not have occurred in the absence of the HIV epidemic. Adding a quarter of TB deaths among HIV-negative people to the deaths directly attributable to HIV/AIDS suggests that HIV/AIDS will be responsible for about one-fifth of all infectious disease deaths in low-income countries in the year 2020.

AIDS usually strikes prime-age adults, often people who are raising children and are at or near the peak of their income potential, because it is sexually transmitted. In the absence of AIDS, prime-age adults tend to be less vulnerable to sickness and death than children, adolescents, or old people. Accordingly, AIDS casts an even larger shadow on the health of prime-age adults and the welfare of their dependants.

In 1990, HIV was already third after TB and non-TB respiratory infections as a cause of adult death in the developing world; by 2020, HIV will be second only to TB as a killer of prime-age adults in developing countries. Adding one-quarter of TB deaths among HIV-negative prime-age adults makes HIV/AIDS the largest single infectious killer of prime-age adults in the developing world in 2020, responsible for half of all deaths from infectious disease among this important group. The HIV/AIDS share of the adult infectious disease burden varies widely across developing regions.

In Africa, where other infectious diseases decline less quickly than in other regions and HIV/AIDS infection rates are assumed to be levelling off in many areas, HIV/AIDS will 'count for about one-third of these deaths . Because Latin America and the Caribbean countries are projected to make the most progress in reducing other infectious diseases and HIV infection is predicted to continue to rise, HIV will be responsible for almost three-quarters of the infectious disease burden there.

AIDS AND DEVELOPMENT

The health impacts of the disease alone are ample cause for concern. There are additional reasons why the development community in general and policymakers in particular should be concerned about the HIV/AIDS epidemic. First, widespread poverty and unequal distribution of income that typify underdevelopment appear to stimulate the spread of HIV. Second, the accelerated labour migration, rapid urbanisation and cultural modernisation that often accompany growth also facilitate the spread of HIV. Third, at the household level AIDS deaths exacerbate the poverty and social inequality that are conducive to a larger epidemic, thus creating a vicious circle.

Poverty and gender inequality make a society more vulnerable to HIV. The idea that poverty and gender inequality exacerbate AIDS is supported by an exploratory analysis of national level aggregate data on HIV infection rates.

When examining the influence of gender inequality on HIV infection, one must hold constant as much as possible other cultural influences which may be correlated with gender inequality across countries. The first of these, the ratio of mates to females in urban centers, varies remarkably across countries: some countries have fewer male urban residents than female and others have 40 per cent more males.

Other things being equal, one might suppose that commercial sex would be more common in cities where men greatly outnumber women and that HIV levels would therefore be higher. Cities in which men ages 20 to 39 greatly outnumber women do in fact have significantly higher HIV infection rates. For the average country, increasing the job opportunities for young women so that the ratio of mates to females in urban areas falls, for example, from 1.3 to 0.9, would decrease the HIV infection rate by about 4 percentage points.

The second measure related to gender inequality included in the analysis is the gap between adult male and female literacy rates. Again, there is great variation across countries, the literacy rate among men being as much as 25 percentage points higher than among women in some countries. When women are much less literate than men, they may be less able to bargain effectively with men and thus be at greater risk in sexual encounters.

Furthermore, illiterate women will have difficulty finding jobs and thus may depend more on sexual relationships for economic survival, again reducing their bargaining power.

Economic growth and AIDS

A country that improves per capita income and reduces inequality, for example, by implementing investment policies that generate jobs and raise economic growth, will reduce its risk of suffering an AIDS epidemic or help to minimize an epidemic already under way. If, in addition, the country acts to close the literacy and urban employment gaps between men and women, HIV would have even more difficulty spreading. Unfortunately, some of the very processes that might achieve these goals can also stimulate the spread of AIDS. And other policies that sometimes accompany growth, without necessarily contributing to it, can likewise worsen the epidemic.

Some studies have suggested that immigration itself contributes to economic growth. This would hardly be surprising, since immigrants are often among the hardest-working and most enterprising people in any country. However, a cross-country regression analysis suggests that countries with larger immigrant populations tend to have larger AIDS epidemics: other things being equal, a country in which 5 per cent of the population is foreign- born can expect to have an infection rate about 2 percentage points higher than a country with no foreign-born.

If immigration is beneficial to economic growth, reducing immigration may slow it, a result that, in addition to many other negative effects, may stimulate the spread of AIDS. Attempting to screen out HIV-positive immigrants is unlikely to be very effective, since immigrants are more likely to become infected after they have arrived in a new country, when they are disconnected from the social networks of their former homeland than before leaving home.

Economic development projects that do not generate sufficient net economic returns after covering the cost of mitigating negative impacts, including the spread of AIDS, should be rejected as undesirable—even if the gross returns are quite large. Sometimes a low-income society beginning rapid growth may face an increased risk of AIDS as a result of a broad shift from conservative social norms to more liberal attitudes; these attitudes often include greater individual freedom, especially for women.

Controlling for all other variables described above, a high degree of social conservatism is associated to a statistically significant degree with lower rates of HIV infection. This does not necessarily imply that governments should attempt to instill or maintain social conservatism simply to minimize HIV; such broad social values may in any event be very difficult for governments to shape.

However, the evidence does suggest the usefulness of an explicit government education policy that would help young people entering a rapidly modernising society to recognise and avoid risky sexual encounters. A final factor in the regression analysis that is not associated with development but can be readily affected by government policy is the level of militarisation.

Net macroeconomic impact

HIV/AIDS is spreading rapidly and is virtually always fatal. It will significantly reduce population growth and economic growth. Populations in badly hit countries will decline in absolute terms and that there will be an associated collapse in economic output. However, the available evidence suggests that the impact of AIDS on these variables, although varying across countries, will generally be small relative to other factors. Moreover, at a very crude level, declines in population growth due to HIV/AIDS will tend to offset declines in economic growth, so that the net impact on gross domestic product (GDP) growth per capita will generally be small. HIV/AIDS is expected to reduce population growth rates in many countries, but in no country is an absolute decline in population expected. The latest projections suggest that declines in population growth rates from HIV/AIDS mortality will range from about 0.1 percentage point in Thailand to 2.3 percentage points in Botswana and that the median country's population growth rate will decline by about 1 percentage point.

Over time, such a reduction in growth would result in a significantly smaller population than would have existed in the absence of AIDS. In Zambia, for example, the population is predicted to be 7 per cent smaller in 2005 than it would have been without AIDS. In two countries with very severe AIDS epidemics, Botswana and Zimbabwe, the projections suggest that by 2010 the population will cease growing.

The impact of AIDS on economic growth is a much more complex issue than the impact on population growth. The inadequacy of GDP per capita as a measure of human welfare is striking when changes in per capita GDP are used to measure the impact of AIDS. Other things held constant, the death of people with higher incomes will reduce average income—even though the welfare of those who remain alive has not changed.

Conversely, the death of those with lower incomes raises average income, without necessarily improving the lot of any surviving individual and despite the suffering and economic losses of the families of those who died. Further, increased spending on health care and funerals is included in GDP calculations. As a result, per capita GDP may increase, even though overall well-being has not improved and the incomes of survivors have been reduced. With these caveats in mind, it is nonetheless possible to estimate the size of the epidemic's impact on individual incomes.

This impact will depend on characteristics of the country, including the severity of the epidemic, the efficiency of the labour market, the proportion of the treatment cost of AIDS financed from savings, the distribution of HIV infection by productivity of worker, the time lost from work by the person with AIDS and others as a result of his or her sickness and the effectiveness of household and community formal and informal insurance mechanisms. Because AIDS kills prime-age adults, many of whom are at the peak of their economic productivity, the shock of AIDS to the labour market is one mechanism through which AIDS might affect growth.

However, in economies with substantial unemployment, firms should find it easy replace sick or deceased workers, particularly if they are not key personnel. Other things being equal, the impact of the AIDS epidemic will be small until the economy begins to grow and is constrained by labour supply rather than by insufficient demand.

Another factor that is likely to have a significant effect on the size of the macroeconomic impact of the epidemic is the percentage of AIDS treatment costs financed from savings. Since spending on AIDS treatment is likely to reduce the capital available for more productive investment, the higher the proportion of care financed from savings, the larger the reduction in growth resulting from the epidemic. If one takes these factors into consideration, a rough estimate would be that a generalised epidemic, would reduce per capita GDP by as much as half a percentage point per year.

In some very poor sub-Saharan African countries, growth rates in GDP per capita that are already negative may deteriorate even further as a result of the AIDS epidemic. But some countries with severe AIDS epidemics, including Botswana, Thailand and Uganda, have been growing rapidly. With per capita growth rates in excess of 5 per cent per year, a reduction of 0.5 per cent in per capita growth will not be crippling. For these countries, as for many other countries where the epidemic may peak at lower infection levels, the more serious consequences will be the impacts on public health spending and on poverty.

The macroeconomic effects of AIDS are likely to be small in most countries, but, severely affected countries will experience quite large impacts on their health sector and on the poor. The effect on the health sector will be to increase the price and reduce the availability of health care for everyone, which will tend to hurt the poor most. Furthermore, among the households that suffer an AIDS death, lower-income households will be less able than others to cope with the medical expenses and other impacts, including loss of income.

One important way in which AIDS is likely to exacerbate poverty and inequality—and indeed, one of the most tragic effects of the epidemic—is the increase in the number of children who lose one or both parents. To be sure, AIDS is not the only cause of orphanhood: in some countries other causes of prime-age adult death may orphan many more children than AIDS. Nonetheless, as AIDS mortality rises, growing numbers of children will be orphaned by the disease.

GOVERNMENT ROLE IN CONFRONTING AIDS

The need for governments to confront the epidemic appears straightforward. For many people the human suffering caused by the epidemic is reason enough for governments to be involved. However, there are other important reasons for government involvement, some of which are not so readily evident. Analysis of these rationales for government involvement is a necessary foundation for considering how governments should confront HIV/AIDS.

One economic rationale for government involvement in HIV prevention is very straightforward: prevention is much cheaper than treatment and avoids the sickness and death that are the final outcome of the disease. This argument is particularly important in the many low-income countries where governments remain committed to publicly financed curative health care. In such countries, the high cost of AIDS treatment starkly reveals the scarcity of resources.

As the number of AIDS cases and treatment costs mount, it becomes painfully evident that AIDS treatment is consuming public resources that could have been used for other human needs. Yet governments may find it very difficult to restrict financing for AIDS treatment without at the same time reassessing their commitment to publicly financed health care. Indeed, in many countries there are political pressures to subsidise AIDS treatment at a higher level than other health care services and these pressures are likely to grow as the number of people with HIV increases. For all these reasons, a government that wishes to continue subsidising health care should initiate aggressive prevention efforts as early in the epidemic as possible. Even governments that are attempting to reduce subsidies for curative care would do well to invest in HIV prevention, since political pressures for subsidised care may be very difficult to resist.

Public economics rationale for governments

A government does not subsidise curative health care and

that it is able to resist all pressures to do so. Given that HIV/AIDS is primarily transmitted by sex, would there still be a rationale for government intervention to reduce its spread? The answer from a public economics perspective is yes. To understand why, it is useful to first consider the public economics rationale for government intervention against other contagious diseases, such as TB. If all markets worked perfectly, governments would not need to be involved in the fight against these diseases. Instead, each person at risk of infection would pay an appropriate share of the cost of reducing his or her risk.

In reality, of course, there is no mechanism other than government through which individuals can pay this amount. Since a person infected with TB is likely to consider only the benefits to himself when deciding whether to pay for treatment, without government intervention people infected with TB would be cured less often than everyone else would prefer. Economists call the benefits of treatment that are not captured by the person paying for the treatment external benefits and the negative impacts on others of not getting treatment external costs. These externalities, if large, are a strong economic justification for government intervention.

In giving advice on how governments should spend scarce public resources, economists look for evidence of large externalities or public goods. Where these exist, markets are said to have failed and public intervention to address the market failure is warranted. In the case of TB, malaria and other diseases that may strike people regardless of their individual behaviour, the public economics arguments for government intervention due to market failure are clear. At first consideration, it may appear that externalities and public goods are not a significant concern in the case of STDs, including HIV. Since most STD transmission occurs as a result of a voluntary act between two people, each can weigh his or her risk and proceed only if the benefits of doing so outweigh the risks. The problem, of course, is that the decision of these two people has consequences for many others, endangering marital sex and procreation as well as more casual sexual relationships.

In public economics terms, there are external benefits associated with refraining from risky sex. Since an individual cannot capture these benefits, he or she will be less prudent than would otherwise be the case. The result: higher STD infection rates and a greater risk of infection for everyone who is sexually active, even those who are monogamous, since most people cannot be sure that their partner is also monogamous. In such a situation, government intervention is justified if it can increase the incentives for the most sexually active individuals to practice safer sex (or for injecting drug users to adopt safer injecting behaviour) to the point that their decisions more closely reflect consideration for the social consequences of risky behaviour.

The arguments above for government intervention to prevent the spread of STDs apply even more strongly to HIV/AIDS. In addition to being sexually transmitted, HIV/AIDS has two characteristics that worsen the market failures associated with the disease—and suggest that governments should be particularly concerned about HIV prevention. The most obvious is that AIDS cannot be cured and is almost always fatal.

Since individuals have little control over their exposure to TB and since people who have HIV and TB can spread TB even to people who are HIV-negative, the link between HIV and TB further strengthens the arguments for a government role in controlling HIV. While this link suggests that HIV/AIDS should receive special attention, the close epidemiological relationship between HIV and other STDs, means that in practice any effective strategy against HIV will almost certainly involve stepped-up prevention efforts against other STDs and vice versa.

Since the monitoring problem described above applies equally to all STDs, governments would have a role in STD control even in the absence of HIV. Because HIV multiplies manyfold the external costs associated with a case of gonorrhoea or genital ulcer disease, the presence of HIV strengthens the argument for government intervention to control the spread of all STDs.

Government role in generating information

In some countries, HIV/AIDS has now been present for two decades, long enough for most people to know that it adds a mortal risk to sexual liaisons; yet surveys show that an alarmingly large proportion of people in some countries still do not know how to protect themselves. In other societies, the disease is still new, an invisible danger spreading through an unsuspecting citizenry that, because of HIV's two-to-twenty-year asymptomatic period, has yet to be jolted by a sudden upsurge in AIDS deaths. In either society, only the government has the incentives and the capacity to generate the information that permits people to take the first steps toward self-protection. Information about the state of the epidemic and how to avoid infection is a true public good.

Although it is possible to restrict access to information, for example, by selling it in magazines available only to subscribers, valuable information has a tendency to spread beyond those to whom it is sold. Therefore, private firms have less incentive to produce and sell information and will produce less of it than is socially desirable. This is particularly true of information from epidemiological monitoring of infection rates in various groups in society.

The value of public health surveillance lies in announcing the results, so that people are aware of the disease in their midst and can take steps to protect themselves by reducing risky behaviour. The public role in the production of new information reaches beyond monitoring the epidemic to include various types of research that enable a more effective response.

In all countries, governments will require country-specific information about how to identify and reach people at highest risk of becoming infected and spreading HIV to others. Research that improves the effectiveness of interventions throughout the country has important public good qualities and therefore deserves government support. Some information relevant to prevention efforts, including biomedical insights into the virus, is an international public good.

AIDS AND HUMAN RIGHTS

HIV/AIDS has created new human rights concerns and cast harsh new light on long-standing problems. Thus, the universally recognised obligation of governments to protect people from harm at the hands of others is a compelling reason for governments to play an important role in society's response to HIV. Because people can be infected with HIV and transmit it to others for years before they become ill, the disease defines and creates a new minority group in society. Government responses to the difficult task of balancing the interests of the infected against the interests of others have varied widely.

The human rights rationale for a government role related to HIV/AIDS is dramatic and unambiguous in instances where sexual relations are compelled by force. Here the government's overarching responsibility in protecting individuals from physical harm and forced exploitation is reinforced by the public interest in preventing the spread of HIV.

POLITICS AND AIDS

Politics and social norms make designing and implementing effective AIDS policies uniquely challenging. The specific problems and their solutions will vary across countries. Nonetheless, four types of issues have commonly arisen:

- — denial that HIV/AIDS may be a problem
- — reluctance to help people who practice risky behaviour to avoid infection
- — preference for moralistic responses
- — pressure to spend on treatment, at the expense of prevention.

Denial is typically seen at the earliest stages of the epidemic, when the long asymptomatic period of the disease makes its effects nearly invisible. An extreme form of denial includes unwillingness to acknowledge that extramarital sex and illicit drug use exist in the society. Some officials in societies with conservative social mores may be genuinely unaware of the extent of extramarital sex or illicit drug use; the more conservative the society, the greater the likelihood that such activities are clandestine.

More typically, officials may be aware of such activities but lack information to evaluate their relevance to the AIDS threat In such a situation, officials concerned about the possible negative reaction of their constituents may be reluctant to initiate the frank, public discussion that could provide the basis for formulation and implementation of an effective HIV prevention program.

In some instances, officials may acknowledge that HIV/AIDS poses a threat to society but nonetheless may be reluctant to advocate HIV prevention programs that focus directly on the people most likely to contract and spread the disease: sex workers, injecting drug users, male homosexuals and bisexuals with many partners and others with high rates of sexual partner change. Although such approaches are most cost-effective—they may be impeded by two types of forces.

On one hand, politicians and policymakers responding to the vast majority of their constituents, who do not engage in high-risk behaviour, may feel little pressure to focus prevention programs on those most likely to contract and spread HIV. This is because few constituents are likely to understand the links between infection rates in people practising high-risk behaviour and their own risk of infection. On the other hand, to the extent that people engaged in high-risk activities have political influence, they or their advocates may oppose prevention efforts focused on themselves, out of concern that such programs will fuel discrimination.

Given the lack of demand for prevention programs for those practising high-risk behaviour from the majority of their constituents and resistance from those who would be the primary beneficiaries of such programs, officials may find it easier to initiate a general public information campaign, even if this is less likely to reach those most apt to contract and spread the disease. Even if politicians and policymakers get past denial and the reluctance to target prevention interventions to those with the riskiest behaviour, some interventions may well have broader social support than others.

In many societies, encouraging abstinence from extra-marital sexual relations or from injecting drug use would be widely viewed as morally correct, while providing free condoms for sex workers and their clients and offering clean needles to injecting drug users would be regarded by many people as facilitating immoral activity.

SELECTED READINGS

Albert Jovell, "The Social Dimension of AIDS" (Sociology Department, Autonomous University of Barcelona, 1990) (Mimeo).

Dennis Altman, *The Homosexualization of America,* Boston: Beacon Press, 1982.

Dorothy Nelkin and Stephen Hilgartner, "Distributed Dimensions of Risk: A Public School Controversy Over AIDS," *Milbank Quarterly*, Supplement 1 (1986).

Joseph Lopez, "The Children of AIDS, the Sad Consequence of a Disease," *La Vanguardia* (March 7, 1990), 4-5 ("Health and Quality of Life" supplement).

Ministry of Health, AIDS Reports, Madrid, Ministry of Health, 1989.

"Recommendations for Preventing Transmission of Infection with Human T-Lymphotropic Virus Type III/Lymphadenopathy-Associated Virus," *MMWR* (November 11, 1986).

The World Health Organisation (WHO), in 1991, predicted 20 million cases of AIDS by the end of the century.

Bibliography

Aina, T.A., 1991, Patterns of Bisexuality in Sub-Saharan Africa. In: *Bisexuality and HIV/AIDS: A Global Perspective*, edited by R. Tielman, M. Carballo, and A. Hendriks, Bufallo, NY: Prometheus Books.

Albert Jovell, "*The Social Dimension of AIDS*" (Sociology Department, Autonomous University of Barcelona, 1990) (Mimeo).

Alfonso Delgado Rubio, "*AIDS Manual: Medical and Social Aspects*", Mandrid: Organisation Medica Colegial, 1987.

American Academy of Pediatrics Policy Statement. "Breast-feeding and the Use of Human Milk". *Pediatrics*, 1997.

American Psychiatric Association 1994, *Diagnostic and Statistical Manual of Mental Disorders* (4th Ed.) (DSM-IV). Washington, DC: Author.

Antoni, M., Schneiderman, N., Klimas, N., LaPerriere, A., Ironson, G., & Fletcher, M. 1991, "*Disparities in psychological, neuroendoctrine, and immunologic patterns in asymptomatic HIV-1 seropositive and seronegative gay men*". *Biological Psychiatry*.

Antonucci, T. C. (1989), Social support influences on the disease process. In L. L. Carstensen & J. M. Neale (eds.), *Mechanisms of psychological influence on physical health, with special attention to the elderly*. New York: Plenum Press.

Bandura, A. (1994), Perceived self-efficacy in the exercise of control over AIDS infection. In: V. M. Mays, G. W. Albee, & S. F. Schneider (Eds.), *Primary Prevention of AIDS: Psychological Approaches*. Newbury Park, CA: Sage.

Barlett, J. G. (1993), *The Johns Hopkins Hospital guide to medical care of patients with HIV infection*. Baltimore, MD: Williams & Wilkins.

Boyd-Franklin, N., Aleman, J. del C., Jean-Gilles, M. M., & Lewis, S. Y. (1995). Cultural sensitivity and competence. In N. Boyd-Franklin, G. L. Steiner & M. G. Boland (Eds.), *Children, families and HIV/AIDS*. New York: Guilford Press.

Bridbord K., Willoughby A. "Vitamin A and mother-to-child transmission". *Lancet*, 1994.

Broadhead, W. E., Kaplan, B. H., James, S. A., Wagner, E.H., Schoenbach, V. J., Grimson, R., Heyden, S., Tibblin, G., & Gehlbach (1983), "Reviews and commentary: The epidemiologic evidence for a relationship between social support and health". *American Journal of epidemiology*.

Burgess, A. P., Irving, G., & Riccio, M. (1993), "The reliability and validity of a symptom checklist for use in HIV infection: A preliminary analysis". *International Journal of STD & AIDS*.

Campbell, C. A. (1990), Prostitution and AIDS. In D. G. Ostrow (ed.), *Behavioural aspects of AIDS*. New York: Plenum Press.

Carmen, E., & Brady, S. M. (1990). AIDS risk and prevention for the chronic mentally ill. *Hospital and Community Psychiatry*.

Catania, J. A., Turner, H. A., Choi, K., & Coates, T. J. (1992). "Coping with death anxiety: Help-seeking and social support among gay men with various HIV diagnoses". *AIDS*.

Cockerell, C. J. (1992), Cutaneous and historic signs of HIV infection other than Kaposi's sarcoma. In G. P. Wormser (ed.), *AIDS and other manifestations of HIV infection*. New York: Raven Press.

College of Health, *AIDS and the Government* (London: College of Health, 1986).

Datta P, Embree JE, Kreiss JK, et. al., "Mother-to-child transmission of human immunodeficiency virus" type 1: report from the Nairobi study. *Journal of Infectious Diseases*, 1994.

Dennis Altman, The Homosexualization of America, Boston: Beacon Press, 1982.

Department of Health (Cox Report), *Short-term Predictions of HIV and AIDS in England* (London: HMSO, 1988); N. Wells, the AIDS Virus: Forecasting its Impact (London: Office of Health Economics, 1986).

Dorothy Nelkin and Stephen Hilgartner, "Distributed Dimensions of Risk: A Public School Controversy Over AIDS," *Milbank Quarterly*, Supplement 1 (1986).

Dunn DT, Newell ML, Ades AE, Peckham C. "Risk of human immunodeficiency virus type 1 transmission through breast-feeding". *Lancet*, 1992.

"Education and Foster Care of Children Infected with Human T-Lymphotropic Virus type III/Lymphadenopathy Associated Virus," *MMWR* (August 30, 1985).

Finley, J. L., Joshi, V. V., & Neil, J. S. A. (1992), General pathology of HIV infection. In G. P. Wormser (ed.) *AIDS and other manifestations of HIV infection*. New York: Raven Press.

Fischl, M. A. (1992), Treatment of HIV infection. In M. A. Sande & P. A. Volberding (eds.), *The medical management of AIDS*. Philadelphia: Saunders.

Fox, R., Odaka, N., Brookmeyer, R., & Polk, B. F. (1987), "Effect of HIV antibody disclosure on subsequent sexual activity in homosexual men". *AIDS*.

Gochros, H. L. (1992), "The sexuality of gay men with HIV infection". *Social Work*.

Gordon, G., and T. Klouda. 1989. *Preventing a Crisis: AIDS and Family Planning Work*: London: International Planned Parenthood Federation.

Greenberg BL, Semba RD, Vink P. et. al. "Vitamin A deficiency and maternal-infant transmission of HIV in two metropolitan areas in the United States". *AIDS*, 1997.

Gupta, S., Anderson, R., & May, R. (1989), "Networks of sexual contacts: Implications for the pattern of Spread of HIV". *AIDS*.

Hackl, K., Kalichman, S. C., & Somlai, A. (1995, February). *Women with HIV/AIDS: The dual challenges of patient and primary caregiver*. Conference on HIV infection in Women, Washington, DC.

Hope, A.S., Timmel and P. Hodzi. 1984. *Training for Transformation: A Handbook for Community Workers*. Gweru, Zimbabwe: Mambo Press.

House, J. S., Landis, K. R., & Umberson, D. (1988), "Social relationships and Health". *Science*.

Jillson-Boostorm, I. (1992), The impact of HIV on minority

populations. In P.I. Ahmed & N. Ahmed (Eds.), *Living and dying with AIDS*. New York: Plenum Press.

Joseph Lopez, "The Children of AIDS, the Sad Consequence of a Disease," *La Vanguardia* (March 7, 1990), 4-5 ("Health and Quality of Life" supplement).

Levine, C., & Stein, G. (1994). *Orphans of the HIV epidemic*. New York: The Orphan Project.

Linn, J. G., Lewis, F. M., Cain, V. A., & Kimbrough, G. A. (1993), "HIV-illness, social support, sense of coherence, and psychosocial well-being in a sample of help-seeking adults". *AIDS Education and Prevention*.

M. Pollak, "AIDS policy in France: Biomedical Leadership and Preventive Impotence," in Action on *AIDS: National Policies on Comparative Perspective*.

Markowitz, J. C., Klerman, G. L., & Perry, S. W. (1993), "An interpersonal psychotherapeutic approach to depressed HIV-seropositive patients". In W. H. Sledge & A. Tasman (eds.), *Clinical challenges in psychiatry*. Washington, DC: American Psychiatric Press.

Miller, D. & Riccio, M. (1990), Editorial review: Non-organic psychiatric and psychosocial syndromes associated with HIV-1 infection and disease. *AIDS*.

Miller, J. E. (1983), Coping with chronic illness. In J. F. Miller (ed.), *Coping with chronic illness: Overcoming powerlessness*. Philadelphia: Davis.

Miller, R. L., Holmes, J. M., & Auerbach, M. I. (1992, August), "*Volunteer experiences of providing AIDS-related educational services*". Paper presented at the 100th Annual Convention of the American Psycho-logical Association, Washington, DC.

Ministry of Health, *AIDS Reports*, Madrid, Ministry of Health, 1989.

Naficy, A. B., & Soave, R. (1992), Cryptosporidiosis, isosporiasis, and microsporidiosis in AIDS. In G. P. Wormser (ed.), *AIDS and other manifestation of HIV infection*. New York: Raven Press.

Nduati R, John GC, Mbori-Ngacha DA, et. al., "Breast disease among lactating HIV-1 infected women". *Xth ICASA*. Abidjan.

Nicolosi, A., Leite, M. L., Musicco, M., Arici, C., Gavazzeni, G., & Lazzarin, A. (1994). "The efficiency of male-to-female and female-to-male sexual transmisstion of the human immunodificiency virus: A study of 730 stable couples". Epidemiology.

Oaklander, V. (1998). *Windows to our children*. Highland, NY: Center for Gestalt Development.

Obbo, C., 1993. HIV Transmission Through Social and Geographical Networks in Uganda. *Social Science and Medicine*.

Office of Technology Assessment, the Public Health Service's Response to AIDS (Washington, D.C.: Government Printing Office, 1985): *The National Academy of Science, Confronting AIDS: Update 1988*, Washington, D.C.: National Academy of Science Press, 1988.

Ostrow, D., Joseph, J., Kessler, R., Soucy, J., Tal, M., Eller, M., Chmiel, J., & Phair, J. (1989), "Disclosure of HIV antibody status: Behavioural and mental health correlates". *AIDS Education and Prevention*.

Ozawa, M., Auslander, W., & Slonim-Nevo, V. (1993), "Problems in financing the care of AIDS patients". *Social Work*.

Padian, N. S., (1988), "Preventing the heterosexual spread of AIDS". *Journal of the American Medical Association*, 1879.

Pfeiffer, N. (1992, October), "Long term survival and HIV disease: The role of exercise and CD4 response in HIV disease". *AIDS Patient Care*.

Piette, J. D., Thompson, B. J., Fleishman, J. A., & Mor, V. (1993). The organisation and delivery of AIDS case management. In V. J. Lynch, G. A. Lloyd, & M. Fimbres (Eds.), *The changing face of AIDS: Implications for social work practice*. Westport, CT: Auburn House.

Potts, M., Anderson, R., & Baily, M. C. (1991), Slowing the spread of human immunodeficiency virus in developing countries. *Lancet*.

"Pneumocystis Pneumonia-Los Angles," Morbidity and Morality Weekly Report (June 5, 1991).

Presidential Commission on the HIV Epidemic, Final Report (June 1988), 119.

"Recommendations for Preventing Transmission of Infection with Human T-Lymphotropic Virus Type III/Lymphadenopathy-Associated Virus," MMWR (November 11, 1986).

R. Klein and P. Day, "Interpreting the Unexpected: The Case of AIDS Policy Making in Britain," *Journal of Public Policies*.

Robert Holloway, "Lack of Awareness Hurts AIDS Prevention in Japan," *The Daily Yomiuri* (August 11, 1990).

Ronald Bayer, *Private Acts, Social Consequences: AIDS and the Politics of Public Health* (New Brunswick, M. J.: Rutgers University Press, 1991).

Rosenberg, M. J., Holmes, K. K., & the World Health Organization working group on Virucides. (1993), "Virucides in prevention of HIV infection: Research priorities". *Sexually Transmitted Diseases.*

Schoepf, B.G. 1983. Health for Rural Women. *Commurity Action* (Zimbabwe).

Schwartzberg, S. S. (1993), "Struggling for meaning: HIV-positive gay men make sense of AIDS". *Professional Psychology: Research and Practice.*

Sierra Health Foundation (1991). *Challenge for the future: Coordinating HIV/AIDS care and services in the next decade*. Rancho Cordova.

Sikkema, K. J., Kalichman, S. C., Kelly, J. A, & Koob, J. J. Group intervention to improve coping with AIDS-related bereavement: Moel development and an illustrative clinical example, *AIDS Care.*

Slowinski, J. W. (1989, September), "Psychological needs of HIV-positive and AIDS patients". *Medical Aspects of Human Sexuality.*

Somlai, A., & Kalichman, S. (1994, August) *The spiritual practices and needs of people living with IIIV-AIDS.* Paper presented at the 102nd Annual Convention of the American Psychological Association, Los Angeles.

Sweeney, J., Peters, B. S., & Main, J. (1991), "Clinical care and management". *AIDS Care.*

Taerk, G., Gallop, R. M., Lancee, W. J., Coates, R. A., & Fanning, M. (1933), "Recurrent themes of concern in groups for health care professionals". *AIDS Care.*

Thapa S, Short R V, Pott M. "Breast-feeding, birth spacing and their effects on child survival". *Nature,* 1989.

The World Health Organisation (WHO), in 1991, predicted 20 million cases of AIDS by the end of the century.

Thea DM, Steketee RW, Pliner V. et. al., "The effect of maternal viral load on the risk of perinatal transmission of HIV-1". *AIDS*, 1997.

Tross, S., & Hirsch, S. (1988), Psychological distress and neuropsychological complications of HIV infection and AIDS. *American Psychologist.*

Ward-Wimmer, D., and Riley, M. (1991), *Caring at home.* Washington, DC: Child Welfare League of America.

Yates, B., 1982, Colonialism, Education and Work: Sex Differentiation in Colonial Zaire. In: *Women Work in Africa*, edited by E.G. Bay. Boulder, CO: Westview Press.

Index

Acquired Immune Deficiency Syndrome (AIDS), 283
Additional hygiene, 9
Adult death, 21
Adult mortality, 7
Aerosol pentamidine, 264
Aggressive treatment, 3
AIDS control and prevention project, 47
AIDS epidemic, 6
AIDS impact, society in, 1
AIDS, 116
  external control, 121
  internal control, 119
  self-esteem, 121
Antiretroviral (ARV), 2
Antiretroviral medications, 242
Antiretroviral therapies, 258
Assessment data, 211
  convergent, 211
  divergent, 211
Asymptomatic periods, 233

Barre-Sinoussi, Franscoise, 187
Biomedical information, 215
Biomedical interventions, 258
Bisexual men, 181
Blood banks, 11

Casual sex, 104
Chermann, Jean-Claude, 187
Child-spacing effects, 267
Coccidioidomycosis, 250
Cognitive behaviour therapy, 213
Cognitive restructuing , 198
Cognitive restructuring, 214
Colostrum, 272
Commercial sex, 104
Complementary funding, 45
Confidentiality, 224
Contagious diseases, 19
Coping strategies, 124
Cryptococcoses, 250
Cultural modernisation, 288
Cytomegalovirus (CMV), 248
  CMV colitis, 248
  CMV esophagitis, 248
  CMV retinitis, 248

Dideoxycytidine (ddC), 260
Disseminate psychological information, 215
Disulfiram, 263
Domingo, Santo, 101

Electron microscopy, 74
Emotion focused coping, 128
Emotional distress, sign of, 212
Environmental stressors, 167
Enzyme-Linked Immunosorbent Assay (ELISA), 236
Epidemiological relationships, 296

Epstein-Barr virus, 249
Food consumption, 27

Gastrointestinal symptoms, 255
Global Programme on AIDS (GPA), 47
Global survey, HIV for, 76
Gonorrhoea, 19
Gross Domestic Product (GDP), 291
Guinea-Bissau, 72

Hairy leukoplakia, 249
Health product development alliance of, 53
Health promotion, 216
Hematology, 262
Histoplasmosis, 250
HIV antibody testing, 170
HIV antibody, testing of, 167
  bereavement, 175
  gay/bisexual man, 178
  illness-related stressors, 172
  pre-existing social stressors, 178
  social losses, 174
  social stressors, 173
  test result, 170
  urban communities, 179
HIV Baby Booms, 72
HIV infection, 14
HIV infection, coping strategies for, 122
  acceptance/resignation, 127
  avoidance, 128
  cognitive coping strategies, 124
  denial points in, 127
  distraction, 128
  emotional-focused coping, 126
  information seeking, 124
  life-style changes, 125
  medical treatment in, 124
  optimism hope, 129
  optimism/spirituality, 129
  problem-focuses coping, 122
  social activism, 125
  spirituality, 130
HIV infection, developing countries in, 106
HIV negative patients, 13
HIV seropositivity, 217
HIV transmission rates, 62
HIV, epidemiology of, 91
  biology/behaviour, 93
  commercial/casual sex, 102
  concurrent partnerships, 101
  infectiousness, 94
  mixing patterns, 100
  partner change rate of, 99
  serial monogamy, 102
HIV, epidemiology of, 93
Hodgkin's disease, 257
Hospitalisation cost, 5
Human Immunodeficiency Virus (HIV), 284
Human papovavirus, 249
Hypochondriasis, 210

Illness related stressors, 175
Immunologic footprints, 235
Immunologic impairment, 241
Immunology, 262
In utero infection, 269
Infectiousness, duration of, 96
Information seeking, 126
Injecting Drug Use (IDU), 278
Inner city, 182
Inpatient care, 5
International AIDS Vaccine Initiative (IAVI), 54
International community, challenges for, 69

International public good, 297
Intrapartum infection, 269
Isosporiasis, 252

Janeiro, Rio de, 45

Kaposi's sarcoma, 240
Kenyatta National Hospital (KNH), 13

Lymphadenopathy, 232, 250

Macroeconomic impact, 291
Malignancies, 252
Martin, D., 167
Martin, J. L., 176
Mohammad, Mahathir, 60
Mother-to-child transmission (MTCT), 268
Mother-to-child transmission, 3
Multicenter AIDS Cohort Study (MACS), 231
Multifocal leukoencephalopathy, 249
Mycobacterial infections,
Mycobacterium Avium Complex (MAC), 255
Mycobacterium diseases, 254

Naltrexone, 263
Neurology, 262
Neuropsychological effects, 218
Nongovernmental organisations (NGOs), 284
Nongynecologic manifestations, 243

Occupational risk, 10
Oncology, 262
Opportunistic illnesses, 259
Opportunitistic illness, 2

Palliative care, 2
Paulo, Sao, 5
Peer facilitators, 146
Pelvic inflammatory disease, 257
Personal risk assessment, 228
Phosphonosformate, 260
Physical symptomatology, 210
Pneumocystis carinii pneumonia (PCP), 251
Postpartum period, 271
Poverty policy, severe AIDS epidemic in, 30
Pregnant women, 45
Preventing nascent epidemics, 64
Professional caregivers, 139
Progressive Multifocal Leukoencephalopathy (PML), 249
Prophylaxis, 262
Psychometric properties, 208
Public health authorities, 226
Public policy, implications for, 103
Pulmonary tuberculosis, 240, 245

Recurrent bacterial pneumonia, 240, 256
Reed, G.M., 120
Rotating Savings and Credit Associations (ROSCAs), 24

Salmonella infection, 256
Serial monogamy, 104
Serological testing, 235
Severe AIDS
- epidemic, health policy in, 6
- altering household composition, 22
- equal subsidy rates, 16
- humane responses, 18
- increase demand care for, 7
- reduced supply health care, 8

Sex workers, 57
Sexually transmitted disease (STD), 284
Sexually Transmitted Diseases (STDs), 93
Social activism, 127
Social inequality, 289
Social support, functional dimensions of, 138
 emotional support, 142
 HIV infection, 139
 informational support, 143
 instrumental support, 139
 support groups, 141
 volunteer programmes, 146
Social support, structure of, 134
 family support, 136
 friends/peers, 136
 partners relationship, 135
 professional caregivers, 137
Socio-demographic factors, 239
Somatisation, 210
Sress-buffering models, 150
Substance abuse treatment, 219
Syphilis, 19
Syphilis, 257

T-helper lymphocytes, 241
Therapeutic avenues, 262
Toxoplasma gondii, 252
Toxoplasmosis, 252
Triple-drung therapy, 4

Ugandan Blood Transfusion Service, 9

Vegetative symptoms, 207
Vicious circle, 289
Viral infections, 248
Voluntary HIV counselling and testing (VCT), 280
Western AIDS epidemic, rise of, 187
 Bru-Lai samples, 190 Cd4+ cells, 188
 HIV-1 Bru, 187
 Second Bru Cultural (JBB2/LAV), 187
Window period, 272

Zambia, 283
Zidovudine therapy, 259
 toxicity, 260
 treatment, 260